_Auth_

_hoggett1@_
_hotmail.com_

_Tel 0118 9415744_

CW01395236

# FIRST BOOK

# *By John Hoggett*

'One million people commit suicide every year'
**The World Health Organisation**

*John Hoggett*

Published by
Chipmunkapublishing
PO Box 6872
Brentwood
Essex CM13 1ZT
United Kingdom

**http://www.chipmunkapublishing.com**

Edited by: Michele Koh

# FIRST BOOK

First Book (Poetry and Prose)

'Here we are at the poetry reading.

Drinks and eats, passion, glitterati and literati, and a few disaffected young men.

Oh, the Dylan Thomasness of it all.

*John Hoggett*

# FIRST BOOK

## INTRODUCTION

I am a modern beatnik commenting on climate change and child sexual assault. This book is my life and it is not my life. My life has links to the artistic elite of the country and to homeless drug users. I write of homo lust and I paint my nails scarlet in memory of my stepmother's partying.

Climate change threatens us all, oil wars leave many shaken, and drug companies continue to sell brain-damaging drugs to the distressed.

These are the writings of a slightly distressed man who never got offered psychiatric drugs but instead found poetry and performance and now publication. This is the better option.

*John Hoggett*

# FIRST BOOK

## A CYNIC'S TALE - THE ETERNAL TRIANGLE

Once there was a wimp who wouldn't say boo to a goose. He was called Wally. Now Wally knew he was a wimp so he wore a badge that said, 'please don't hit me,' - it was very small and people had to peer over him to read it, pinned on the lapel of his now rather small school blazer (actually it was his sister's, his mum had thrown his away years ago).

A lot of people were so confused or disgusted by this badge that they turned away in confusion and disgust, obvious really. Wally despised them for not appreciating his honesty and then thought of them as inferior beings - he felt very lonely.

Lots of people picked at Wally and he got small - or perhaps he stooped a lot. Nobody hit him though - it was no fun; he was such a wally and never fought back. Finally, a mentally deficient zomboid called Martin socked Wally good and hard one day. Martin was lookin' for a fight and would have socked a soggy cabbage from yer average canteen dinner if he couldn't find a real person to fight - or even a Wally.

Our hero, Wally you git, not that psychotic ape Martin (please excuse that last metaphor, I'm sure apes are generally quite nice animals) cowered - shivered - snivelled - looked away, looked at the descending fist, looked away gain - took a big deep breath and changed before our very eyes into an Avenging Angel, righting the wrongs of all wimps, past and present. He stood upright drew back his paw and laid Martin out. Kicking him in the bollocks for good measure.

Wally was jubilant. Martin was in casualty receiving treatment for damages received to his genitalia (how embarrassing, he didn't know where to put his eyes). Wally got cool. Went to Top Man for new gear, went to Vidal's for a new Barnet, polished up his shoes and went out on the town. Knockin' 'em down -the drinks that is. Never a frown. Hi jinx - lots of stinks, sex and love and never drew blood. Our all American Hero.

He had a hobby too. Saving Women from embarrassing and painful situations. He escorted many a battered wife to Women's Aid, or at least as near as was allowed, by common consent. He listened to their break-ups, both marital and psychotic. His ear was always there to be bent. His shoulder an ever present support for the female population's problems. Year after year Wally did what he could - childcare, counselling and company were his watchwords. And, if he couldn't help, he would suffer along side, in a slightly distorted belief that 'a trouble shared is a trouble halved'.

Then one day people started to notice Wally's spirits flagging. His ear was not so attentive, his shoulder started to crumble, some women found that hugs from Wally turned to suppressed sobs and they weren't sure if they should be giving the hugs instead.

Wally retired to bed-sit land.


## WHO AM I?

Time for a personality transplant don't you think? I think so. What about this one? Something to try out for an entertaining few days with a small group of semi-strangers in Bologna, Cornwall or Hay-on Wye.

Female, Mid-Atlantic, long auburn hair, piled in artful disarray that took three-quarters of an hour, with gel, hair drier, mousse and at least three mirrors. Nice, not too long, scarlet nails, though we won't be vulgar enough to call them scarlet, rather some frenchified, arty name that implies sophistication, but with that graceful touch of accessibility, say Debussy or Rouge-et-Roué?

She is graceful, charming and takes gentle pride in mocking other's pride, in a genteel and confident manner, with a laugh that hints at Champagne. Trapped in the body of a gay man she makes the best of things, the only thing possible in the circumstance.

This veneer of charm hides - nothing. She possesses a billowing cerise dress that one of Charlie's Angels might have worn to a cocktail party, thrown on a yacht by some foreign Prince. In her head, beneath the charm, the dress, nails and artfully cascading hair is - nothing. Oh, a knowing hold on the pomposity of others, men in particular, but no central being. No juiciness, danger, intrigue, deep philosophy, sense of wonder, bitter tears or the indulgence of occasional dumpiness. No. Full but shallow is the explanatory phrase here.

We love her. She comes in useful so often, a boon to every party. Such knowingness, such aplomb, but friendly too. If you like that sort of thing, and mainly, we do.

## POEMS - BY EXCUSE

I'm Bored!
I'll write a poem,
It'll kill the time
And maybe,
I can read it to someone.
Maybe I can get it published,
And be famous.
Boredom and frustration
To Fame and Fascination.
The working class had punk
But I'll have publication.
Now which is more worthwhile
I ask myself?

# FIRST BOOK

## BREAD

The food of life,
The stuff of life.
I like mine brown - wholemeal,
Nothing too heavy
But good and plain, peasant food.
A fitting background to every meal.
Nothing too fancy, but nourishing and wholesome.
Come share some with me,
If not the crust, perhaps not the crumb,
But come then, let us celebrate - bread.


## UNTITLED 1

Mother and child
　Mary mild,
　　Smile on me sweetly
　　　As the sun shines gently.
　　　　The garden is glorious
　　　　　But the gardener lugubrious,
　　　　　　Frown on the flowers
　　　　　　　As the snapdragon glowers.

*John Hoggett*

## UNTITLED 2

Powerful intoxicants,
   Sweet scented mendicants.
    Broom flowers shimmering,
     Parlour dried Hippie thing.
    Youthful exuberance
      To later day Petulance.
     A middle aged frown
       Regrets gullible clown.

## HELLO

Sleep
Sleepy
Sleepers
Sleeping
Sleep
Goodnight.

## JUVENILIA

A small day,
A wet life,
A drippy boy.

# FIRST BOOK

## IMPERFECT POEM

Sometimes I wake up and I think,
'I wish my mother were dead'.
Then I imagine helping her on her way.
I role over, hit the pillow, rub my tummy,
        shout out and get up.
I go and buy strong coffee
        and bananas and I have breakfast.
The day rolls on and this is my life.

## THE BUSINESS

Some mothers, need to study.
Some mothers should go to school.
Some mothers need to learn a bit
Of home economics of the soul.

Some fathers, don't deserve the title.
Some fathers, shouldn't live at home.
I think, they are merely sperm donors,
And I would like to see them
        2,000 miles away,
Available in emergency, by fax or
        maybe answer phone.

## TENDER TRAPS

Burn Baby Burn
My body's on fire.
You scorched me with your touch,
Your touch is like fire lighters.
So I'll put me in the water
And I'll see you in the fire grate.
I'll get out of my hell
And I'll see you in yours.
So Burn Baby Burn.

## THE EVENT

On a clear summer's day the clear blue sky washes away the memory of her. The soul vampire that raided my groin, my young tender self for her dumb hateful pleasure. And contempt shone in her eyes as I sat on her lap, cringing on the edge of this uncomfortable seat.

Is this a medical examination? If it is I receive no explanation, no healing, no knowledge is gained except to look out for people who say they want to look after me and that disgust and self-loathing is around every corner. Nowhere is safe, least of all home. Trust no one dear, for no one dear to you has your own precious self held high in their esteem.

# FIRST BOOK

And what did she learn? That little boys don't get it up too easily? They respond to contempt? Are frightened by gentle assault, and that assault can be enjoyed? Well listen girl, fuck off and get lost.

Maybe forgetting in this blue blue sky blue bright sky's summer brightness, as I lie in this green field will rest my frightened mind, but maybe it's time to push in that tender face that didn't do it's duty. In the summer clouds I see your face, body and genitals ripped apart as the force of the wind takes it's elemental revenge. Blow wind blow and I will enjoy this sight. Your sinful features painted in white and grey on the pale blue summer sky. Cleanse my soul as my hate is pictured above me whilst yours was wrought on my pale tender body. For I will give it back, this dirt and slime you dumped on me, but meanwhile, I will enjoy your imagined suffering.

Yeah verily, I crave revenge.

## THOUGHT

'I live in flash back city'

## THE CIRCUS

Mama, take me to the circus,
For I would like to see the acrobats.
See them perform and jump through hoops,
As I do for you.
But perhaps the price
Will be cheaper at the circus?
Who knows? For I am not versed
In the rules of money,
And this economy is strange to me.
Why do you need these strange contortions?
And the price we pay is measured in dust.

## COOKING

Mama,
  Take me home from this lonely field
And feed me currants.
  Make me chocolate cake again,
And I will sit at your feet
  On the tiled kitchen floor.
Oh mama bring me home again,
  Bring me home.

# FIRST BOOK

## HEADLINE

Incest Survivor Says,
"For Fuck's Sake Why Can't
You Just Say You Did It
And Have Done With It, Eh?"

## OUT OF THE SUPPORT GROUPS AND INTO THE STREETS.

(Thoughts on the C.R.O.S.S. march - Campaign for the Rights Of Survivors of Sexual Assault - autumn 93)

"Out of the support groups and onto the streets," this could have many meanings. It could mean, that although we may need somewhere confidential and anonymous to talk and cry and rage about the injustices the world has heaped upon us, maybe there comes a time when we need to let the world know about these injustices and to say, "No more.  I will take no more of this shit, we will take no more of it.  Stop these injustices, let us fight them together."

And maybe, "Out of The Support Groups And Into The Streets," means, that although sometimes we may need small groups of intimate friends with whom we will, behind closed doors, share our pain, maybe on days like these why should we not cry, and shake with the fear, and howl with the pain of the injustices heaped upon us. In the streets, in our hundreds and thousands, together.

Let us heal our own and each others pain and in doing so gather the strength to stand up and say we are survivors of child sexual assault. We have been silent long enough. For I will not bear this burden of shame and guilt any more, it was not mine to bear in the first place.

## MAYBE

The Scars And Swipes
Are Not Forever.

## WOULD YOU ADAM AND EVE IT?

God didn't create Adam and Eve he created Adam and Steve! Whoops, is this a slip of the tongue, a slip of the pen or the wishful thinking of a dizzy headed Nancy Queen from Reading? Note; not Queer Tribe member, Poofey Woofter, homosexualist more like. Throw these names and I'll eat 'em up like the Pacmen do.

I saw that fruit and I took a bite, it was crunchy and sweet, juicy with a full, mouth-watering flavour. Would I do it again? Oh yeah, not so often that it palls but yeah. Which brings to mind Ferenzci (maybe this is where bad spelling gets mixed with bad history?) Ferenzci, beloved disciple of Freud gets chucked out of the International Psychoanalytical Association for saying that his clients really have experienced child sexual assault and are not producing some sicko psycho fantasy as Big Daddy Freud said after all.

Ferenzci says:    'CHILD SEXUAL ASSAULT MAKES A PSYCHOLOGIST OF THE CHILD, 'cause Honey, when the bogeyman / woman comes you gotta know what mood they are in and how long this is gonna last. Or maybe you just stared at the wallpaper and noticed how, at this end of the room the seams join perfectly and how at the other end of the room they don't, by maybe half an inch or more, and did you know how fascinating this can be for half to three quarters of an hour at a time?

So the next time you go and see that counsellor or phone up the Samaritans maybe you could wonder how they learn to listen to your every word so carefully and weigh up your silences so succinctly?  Maybe they learnt it the same way I learnt to appreciate the nuances in wallpaper? Why the wallpaper fascination? Well if I did not do that I'd pick up those scissors, turn round and slash a certain persons throat, or not, considering the age and size difference at the time. A whole new meaning to, 'The tree of knowledge'.

Hey Santa Claus, give me a train set instead.

This small twisted fruit is bitter and grieving, learn it well sisters and brothers, with knowledge comes pain, the pain of seeing loved ones hurt and knowing there is nothing you can do about it. Ow! Cast me out of this garden, quick.

## LIVING IN THE AFTERMATH,
## OR, 'I WANT TO BE NORMAL.'

There was a voice
That rolled over my tongue
And out of my mouth.
And it said,
'I want to be Normal,'
And now I realise that I am.
For it is normal
To do strange concoctions of strong
        mind bending drugs.
And normal,
To wear such strange clothes that people
        stare at you in the street.
It is normal to lie in bed,
Screaming in rage and terror,
Two seconds out of every thirty,
Night after night,
Half hours at a time.
It is normal, and indeed natural,
To have cock eyed relationships
With cock eyed men

# FIRST BOOK

Who are as cock eyed as you are.
Where terror and confusion and betrayal
        and countermove,
Intermix with humiliation and threat
And small moments of love.

And normal to have done things
That I choose not to tell you.
Not today, maybe not ever.
For I have my secrets.
And I choose who I tell them to.
For I still have shame.
And that indeed is normal.

And confusion,
And hypocrisy,
And love.

And that, and that too of course, is normal.

# HELP

This is a '**HELP'** card.

To use, present to a passer-by when you are feeling despondent, lonely, or frightened. It may attract someone who is just in the mood to give you their kindness, love, understanding and maybe, even their dinner money. It may attract someone who has gifts that you never knew you needed, and things that you thought useless, that suddenly become wonderful and amazing. It may, therefore, become a '**SERENDIPITY**' card and not a '**HELP**' card at all.

It may, however, attract somebody who thinks they know what you want, and insists on giving it to you, at any cost. If, on displaying your **HELP** card, you attract such a person, may I suggest that you say, "Oh, I'm terribly sorry, what I meant to say is, 'do you have the time?' As I seem to have mislaid my watch.' Then walk, briskly but politely, on.

Discerning between these two types of people can be difficult. Type A can become type B and often does, and vice versa. For the gaining of wisdom can be a long and tortuous path on which I wish you much luck.

From, 'the '**HELP**' fairy'.

___

# FIRST BOOK

## BLUES FOR BABY - A SONG

Sleep and cry my little baby,
Sleep and cry in my arms.
Sleep and cry my little baby,
And I will hold you in my arms.

If there was someone to hold me,
I would cry and I would sleep
But there's no one to hold me,
Never was and never will.

And I will be your manly mother,
In my arms you will lie.
Sleep and cry my manly lover,
I will hold my little one.

In you I see my pain and sorrow,
Sleep and cry in my arms.
In you I hold my pain and sorrow,
Hold myself in loving arms.

Maybe one day I'll go to heaven?
Maybe someone will hold me there?
But I doubt it my little baby,
But I doubt it this very day.

Some day I'll be somebody's baby,
Sleep and cry in his arms.
And he will be my manly lover,
It's my right, I'll live my way.

Now I've found my manly lover,
Sleep and cry in his arms,
And I am his little baby,
Holds me close in lovin' arms.


## BRIEF ENCOUNTER

Close encounter,
Briefly unzipped.
A Glad Grand Manor House
Of an encounter.


## GARDENING

Flower power.
Power flower,
A big gun,
Shooting seeds,
Green and dangerous.


## HAIKU

Shirt buttons undone.
Invitations to caress,
Lightly muscled chest.

# FIRST BOOK

## UNTITLED 4

Chest hair, belly hair,
A swirling mass of sensual patterns.
From nape to naval,
Brush with the grain
Brush against the grain.
Or a tantalising tweak
Of this masculine fun fur.

## UNTITLED 5

```
     A
   FAT        ART
   ART
   MAN
BASTARD       FART
  SHIT
   HEAD       GARTER
   GIT.
```

## WAH!

Bastard Art Man
Trample my Heart.

## DETACHING WITH LOVE

My landscape is peopled by
Distressed, distrustful, despairing,
Dissolute, dumpy dimbos.

Leave them alone and make
Dinner darling, it'll
All come out in the wash.

## CONTRADICTIONS

You know,
    I quite like straight men.
Funny that,
    Kinda' queer, isn't it?

## SOMETIMES

        You know,
Gay men can be quite nice
        Sometimes.

## IDIOT!

To chase the Rainbow,
  The pot of fool's gold at the end of the circle.

# FIRST BOOK

The ever beckoning promise of rest,
It never comes.

For I will not survive
This morning's eternal dream
Of never never land.

And the man who holds your hand
Has scandal writ upon his lips.
I taste betrayal in his constant kiss,
Looks like a man, acts like a puppy dog.
A turncoat when unattended.

---

Put your hand in
my pants lover
and caress me
tenderly for
**I LIKE**      I am scorched
and raw
and in
need
of your
**BEING GAY**   tender
touch to
awaken me
and let my love
of life arise and flow again.

## PRIDE

What is this thing called Pride?
'Tis but the love we have
For ourselves and each other.
The sweat, sex, companionship
And joy, we find in each others lives.
Men with Men
And Women with Women.
Let me roll all over you babe,
And fuck the rest of the world.
Let any of those bastards
Try and stop me loving you,
And their life won't be worth living.
Trust me, hey.

## SHRINKS STINK

Why SHRINKS STINK? Well, psychiatrists look at your symptoms, give you a label and if the label is schizophrenia (something I'm not sure if I believe in) they are likely to give you 'Haldol' also known as 'Haloperidol', a drug which causes irreversible brain damage in up to 50% of the people taking it and whose side effects are deeply disturbing to a lot of the people prescribed it. Psychiatrists often ignore almost everything else about 'schizophrenics,' yet everything about a person affects their state of mind. And as a woman at the C.R.OS.S rally said, 'It is torture to be forced to take these drugs against your wil1 and it is torture to see your friends forced to take these drugs.' (C.R.O.S.S, Campaign for the Rights of Survivors of Sexual Assault).

Most people who see psychiatrists have tragic histories and are not getting on with people in their lives. Drugs may numb you to the criticism you face daily and may suppress the creative element that helps you deal with painful events (though to the outsider your creative resistance may make you appear very strange) but they will not instil a sense of self worth.

What will? In my experience, being with people who have similar experiences, being around an effective political action (whether that be for women's rights, child care, lesbian and gay issues, anti-racist actions, poverty). Just knowing someone is on your side helps; being in an atmosphere where criticism is low; doing what you enjoy with people you like; reviewing painful events with those who are sympathetic; sanctuary from a painful environment whether that be home/work or wherever; help with sorting out practical problems that may have overwhelmed you (e.g. money/housing, food, sexual stuff like worry about H.IV, pregnancy, birth control etc.). Simple sensible stuff really.

Put it this way. If there was a good N.H.S. unit that was for psychiatric patients that are poor women who live with a violent and or alcoholic partner, who have suffered sexual assault, and it used few drugs, it would be swamped. As it is women in such situations may find themselves held in psychiatric hospitals against there will, bored, insulted by staff, forcibly drugged or given E.C.T. (if you want to know what that is like get someone to bang you over the head with a mallet - that will stop you being depressed for a while and no one will know why that works either) and often harassed by male patients.

Or how about queer youth? Young lesbians and gay men have a higher than average rate of attempted suicide. Some may get labelled schizophrenic. After all, when under stress people act strangely and being a gay teenager can be hell. Maybe a subscription to **'SHAVED ANUS'** or **'HORMONE FRENZY'** (gay 'zines) and a label of, 'Oppressed and deeply fucked off,' might help more than injectable Haloperidol and the label, 'psychotic'.

Of course some people go off the deep end and never come back but I think a politicised and supportive environment will help more than anything mainly white, male, heterosexual, middle class psychiatrists have to offer. My local shop keeper is more socially and personally aware than the last psychiatrist I saw. For more on this see **'TOXIC PSYCHIATRY'** by Peter Breggin, Fontana, 1993. Slags off drug treatments, explains various mental states; depression, mania, anxiety, schizophrenic overwhelm etc., promotes drug free treatment and patient led groups - a bit of an anarchist if you ask me.

---

Since writing this piece I found out about, '**New Pin,**' a project for women with young kids who want to learn better parenting skills. It sounds an awful lot like the project that I imagined for, 'Poor women…...'

Newpin is an extraordinarily successful support network, which was launched in Southwark in 1982. Newpin centres are run by the Family Welfare Association

About two thirds of the mothers who come to Newpin are clinically depressed, a third have been sexually or physically abused, a third have been in local authority care. Newpin's work is influenced by Professor George Brown's study on the causes of depression in mothers.

These mothers are overwhelmed by the experience of isolation - but also by the creation of a new network of help and friendship.

Testimony abounds to the confidence Newpin breeds. How do you judge success? By children kept out of care, and away from harm? By parents encouraged to make something of their lives? A former Newpin mother said, "Some people speak of mothers who've gone on college courses, but I think it's a success if a child gets a few extra cuddles."


## IT MUST BE NICE TO HAVE A LOVER

It must be nice to have a lover,
To do the things that lovers do.
I had a lover once,
He would run his fingers through my hair,
I would twist and turn my head,
Massaging his fingers with my hair.
We would lie,
My bum against his tum,
Asleep,
Not asleep,
Sleeping.
And he, when making tea, would turn and say,
        "Sugar?"
I would gently smirk, shake my head and say,
"Surely by now you know, it's been two years."
And he, grinning sheepishly, would turn
To drop the tea bag in the bin.
For theirs was a small well equipped kitchen.
I would often sit there, drinking his tea, holding hands reading the paper.
He would make me Earl Grey, though I prefer Typhoo or even Happy Shopper.
Now he has a different lover, one who neither cares

# FIRST BOOK

For the type or quality of his tea
And I live on my own, sometimes lonely,
sometimes not.
And I think, sometimes, for some of us,
It can be nice to have a lover.

---

I think that those who administer ECT should be
given a shot of their own medicine.

---

## PERSONAL AD

Gay man, moody, short, unemployed, unpopular
git, seeks other for back biting, bitching
relationship. Betrayal especially appreciated, no
violence tolerated, lots of drama assured.

## ON MEN

I was talking to some men who all said they
preferred to talk to women, found it easier to get
support from women. Now that implies that we
don't trust men, are afraid of men and enough fear
will make us angry with men or with ourselves.

Anger with men and fear of men can be expressed
in various ways: putting men down, giving advice,
controlling the conversation, steering it away from
ourselves and personal topics and other ways.

We tell ourselves we don't really hurt, that others are more needy than us, that the men in our lives may appear to be sympathetic, interested and caring but they are not really interested, it is a pretence. This is not to deny that many men are uncaring and inconsiderate but that we do not trust or believe those that are and do them a disservice by not believing them.

We put ourselves down for feeling hopeless, helpless, lonely, sad, frustrated, depressed and needy by saying such things as 'I don't like to moan' and 'Big boys don't cry'. These are all expressions of our fear and lack of trust of men and anger at our own neediness. This is our denial of our hurt and our loneliness and our denial of the loving concern men can have for each other.

Our anger may be expressed in competitiveness, lack of sympathy for others, or in depression.

## I FEEL SICK

And then there was a friend, who said,
'The first time I saw Will and Pete kiss I felt sick.
I forget how much disgust, fear and loathing
Behavior like mine can provoke.
No wonder I feel on edge all the time.
Forget global warming
This town's hot enough already.

# FIRST BOOK

## SOCIAL CONSTRUCT THEORY

When bad things happen to you
There are three choices, we can say:
It is my fault and feel shame, guilt, risk depression,
It is your fault and feel anger, wrath, risk paranoia,
It is chance and feel helpless and very scared.

When good things happen to you
There are three choices, we can say:
I did that and feel proud,
You did that and feel grateful,
It is chance (good luck?) and have a party!

## LONDON'S FLAMES
*(to the tune of London's Burning)*

Oscar Wilde, Oscar Wilde
Joe Orton, Joe Orton
Queer Queer, Queer Queer
Derek Jarman, Derek Jarman.

## FORGIVENESS EXERCISES, SEPTEMBER 94

I forgive nobody, except maybe the cat and then only grudgingly, and I enjoy it, bearing grudges that is.

I forgive myself, actually I did years ago, for being a grumpy git and for sulking a lot.

I forgive myself for loving a violent loony schizophrenic called Martin.

I forgive myself for hating women (well not all of them, or even some of them all of the time but some, sometimes).

I forgive myself for being hurt by Tom's comments about my singing and forgive myself for not telling him.

I forgive myself for getting a hard on while hugging George.

I do not forgive myself for my acts of violence but I hope to understand them more – ah, what the fuck, it happens.

I forgive myself for being nasty to Richard and I forgive him for being a scrawny little unfaithful, moody, envious git who couldn't stand me being good anything in anyone else's eyes and I definitely do not wish that his plane crashes over the Pacific on the way back to New Zealand.

I forgive myself for avoiding Xxxxxx Xxxx (no I'm not going to write his name, what if he read this? What would I have to forgive myself for then eh?).

I'll think about forgiving myself for not seeing my father ever again (maybe?).

I forgive myself, totally, for having no sense of

tune, rhythm or pitch.

I forgive myself for – ouch – I don't forgive myself for <u>that</u>, for consenting to it, yes, for it, no – well maybe I do , I had a part to play but it's all a little complicated and there are other things to think about here.

I forgive myself for not having a job and for not being on a farm by now and for being ill still and for not trusting my health and for not liking my Doctor(s) and for my homeopathic remedies not working enough for my health to be of no bother to me.

I forgive myself my panic attacks and my inability to say things to people and my bitchiness.

But my love of men needs no forgiveness by me or anyone. That would be like forgiving the rain for falling or the sun for shining or the blackberries for growing, small or large, sour or sweet, juicy or full of inedible chewy pips, in good years many and good and in bad years few and desultory. Though I register my disappointment, remembering better years and looking forward to others. Bring on a bumper harvest buster.  Love is a small sweet fruit and so am I.

*John Hoggett*

## FRAGMENT

A passing friend in the night,
A passing park friend in the night
Whose parting lips parted mine.
His beard sliding on my beard;
Like stroking cat fur,
Forward and back forward and back.
He will never be seen again,
He was a passing friend in the night.
A passing park friend in the night,
Whose parting lips parted mine,
Gently, in the night.

## CRUISING PIECE

In that chair sat 'J,' playing piano, well, pleasantly. I stood, amazed; his fingers producing grand chords, and we talked as my hands stroked his back. His face grinning at mine. This warmth I feel like a father's but from someone much more equal, we are equals in this room, at this time, today.

He, at home, is a cycling boy, age 34, in his pianoless council flat, going from green field sex filled man site to green field sex filled man site to home again. A cruising man filling his empty hours with what? Fun, sex and men? I do not know. Love and willies do not always go together for him, but hats he wears. He smiles and frowns,

# FIRST BOOK

and smiles and frowns, and when frowning becomes too much, then off on the bike to those green field sites with woodland hidey – holes where men look like spies, thieves, illicit drug dealers, trading bodies. Is it theirs or yours or mine they trade? Sneaking men of Hampstead, Balham and Holland Park, spies in the houses of love, caught in the act of trading black market goods at prices far higher than they originally imagined. The curse of imprisonment, degradation and shame, though terrible and humiliating, hardly ever comes, though still they dread it, those sneaking men of Balham, Hampstead and Holland Park.

I admire them, I pity them, I loathe and envy them. Hate and incomprehension and longing mix in my heart for them and my heart goes out to 'J,' a man amongst men amongst them, in Hampstead and Balham and Holland Park.

## SALSA DANCE CLASS

His hair is silver blond, well cut
And his teeth smile out like a lighthouse.
Flashing light, but beware of the dark hidden rocks.
He turns, up right, spins again.
I look, enjoy and appreciate.
The lighthouse is there for my safety.
It signals safety, warmth, home, hope, beauty, gives direction.
I navigate a safe distance.
Later I put some money in a collecting tin.
The light says, 'Hidden rocks, keep clear.'
I decide a safe distance and I keep to it,
I carry too much cargo to come in close today.
Rock, hair, smile, lighthouse dancer,
Pretty warnings and noisy nights.
Yes, I'll take care
And sail again on this or some other fortunate sea.


## THE DREAM

He sneezes,
I hand him a handkerchief.
He smiles and wipes his nose.
He places his hand on my shoulder.
I turn, we nuzzle cheeks,
He steps and pecks my lips.
I hold him, hand on shoulder,
He looks in my eyes.

# FIRST BOOK

We kiss,
Sway a little,
Sigh.
We see each other's eyes,
We smile 'till it aches,
I giggle.
He strokes my head,
Smiles,
Steps and turns.
I watch as he leaves the room.
I continue cooking dinner.
He is cleaning the loo.
Yesterday,
I washed underwear,
He cooked dinner,
And tomorrow,
Who knows?


## HIV, SUICIDE, PITY, LIFE AND SELF-SUFFICIENCY

I was thinking of having an HIV test, another HIV test.  My first was two years ago and it was negative, however, there is a slight chance of it having been wrong. I repeat, very slight. Those who wish to know more about the reliability of HIV tests would be advised to go and talk to a knowledgeable health advisor, such as you might find at a GUM clinic or on the National AIDS Helpline – 0800 567123.  Also, since my first test I haven't been exactly celibate, I have indulged in what is euphemistically known as a little low risk activity. Now, do I, in the interest of health education, tell you what that might involve, or do I give in to my natural prudery and draw a veil over it? The latter I think; one can, after all, do too much good work, and we are talking low risk, so if you want to know you'll have to ask someone else.

The reason I am thinking of having another test is because my health is consistently bad with post viral fatigue symptoms, my Doctor is nagging me to have one, and treatments for HIV and associated diseases have improved to such a degree that those of us who want to live and live well are being recommended, more and more, to take the test.

But there's the rub, to live and live well. Do I want to? It might mean a foreseeable end to what has amounted to a somewhat tawdry life. A grateful rest and a long, slow winding down to a peace and magical thinking makes me half believe that a negative state of mind increases the likelihood of a positive test. Of course I romanticise, opportunistic infections associated with AIDS are often painful, frightening, irritating, unsightly and yucky. But where did this idea come from, the idea of slow suicide by nature's hand? Because I take the safer sex message to heart, I don't play Russian Roulette with myself or others. The memory I have is of being sixteen or seventeen, living at

# FIRST BOOK

home with my parents and hearing of someone, possibly someone of my own age, who had cancer. I noted my stepmother and her friends' reaction: pity mixed with concern for this stranger.

Of course I gave no thought to the pain of illness, just the freedom that came with pity. Freedom from the shaming, griping, control of my parents that particularly my stepmother inflicted on me. My father, in the later years of my youth, was mainly disinterested in much about me, except for telling me I was very intelligent, which meant I had to pass lots of exams with good grades. How he knew I don't know, as he never looked at any of my work or much else of what I did with my time.

I thought of being ill as leaving school and living in the tepees in Tepee Valley with my friend Tom Eglestone, a straight-ish youth in the Pre-Raphaelite tradition who I had fallen I love with – ah, the first of many. I had no thought of what being ill would be like, the pain, inconvenience and terror, just that the bonds my parents had placed on me would have no meaning. That surely in their love and pity they would release me and I would grow in freedom as I happily and freely died. In this, 'Love Story,' daydream I gave myself four months.

For me then, freedom, liberty and the desire to be spoilt a little were more important than life, and to some degree still are. So I ask myself how much longer before I am free of these bonds?  For some they are melted in the warm glow of understanding as people mature, forgive each other and talk things over, and some are broken in the hot forge of rage, which seems the route I am slowly taking. For now I realise that we must sometimes fight for the liberty that makes our lives worth living, so I will throw off these shackles and live a little. Keep death for another day, any grateful rest and long slow winding down to peace, will be in the land of the living, and probably in my bed at night. Death can wait and I'll look for a decent life instead, and if I have another HIV test then that is to be dealt with too, whether the result is positive or negative. 'Cause I'm still here, I'm still Queer and I still haven't got enough money to go shopping.

## REVENGE

What else are those violent, car chase, war mongering Rambo movies but the violent revenge fantasies men would like to take out on each other and on women for their early brutalisation? All those early parental injunctions, 'Don't cry,' Well hit him back then,' 'I'm not going to fight your battles for you,' turned to violent fantasies of revenge unconnected with the original event.

Some of us enjoy this, and participate in these images of revenge, others are disgusted by this glorification of male carnage, while some see the justification for their own violence. Rambo as a role model, James Bond as a father or older brother to copy. Michael Ryan learnt a lot from those survivalist magazines.

Nobody knows where my father got the idea of trying to strangle my mother from.

I wonder what would have happened if I had shouted at my Dad, 'Go on then, and don't expect me to visit you in jail when the police drag you off,' or to my step mum, 'Well what do you expect if you treat him like that?' Not quite fair, as their rows were always conducted behind closed doors. Instead, I called my big cousin Chris and after some negotiation they retired, on that Boxing day afternoon some fifteen or so years ago, to the empty bar of the pub they had bought, to discuss, in a slightly more civilised manner, who was to look after and pay for the upkeep of their two children, my half sister and brother, now that my step mother had left my father.  And not even attempted murder, as my father discovered that day, would get her back.

I had stopped my father from strangling my stepmother, and once more found myself looking after other people's interests while no one paid any attention to mine, not even me. Now I take my revenge, apart from the one thousand hours of therapy each year (and my meagre attempts to live well) by writing this book – though cowardice and a certain sensibility stops me from putting my name to it.

## TO ALL YOU VIOLENT MEN

To all you violent men:
Fuck off!
Fuck off back to the womb
And I wish your Dad were sterile.

## UNTITLED 6

'Sometimes I feel so angry I could destroy the planet.'
'Honey, I think maybe someone beat you to it.'

---

If the pen is mightier than the sword, how come those with the nuclear weapons, riot gas and truncheons rule the world?

---

## FRACTAL LOGIC

In, 'right on,' households you can see posters that tell you about whales and Greenpeace's heroic actions to save them. Or pictures of Black heroes, or Goldman, Lenin or Marx, but where are the posters that say the hitting of children is wrong?

# FIRST BOOK

That celebrates the heroes that have fought for children's rights? That say to brutalise the child has the potential for producing a broken spirit or extreme hatred and a need for revenge, which may be carried into adulthood?

Our lives are a mess because we mess up our lives.

The only writing I have seen that makes this clear are the strange garbled artistic writings of the anarchists.

The boss humiliates the man, who goes home to take it out on his wife, who belittles the child who may grow up to take part in cutting the social security system. Simple, simplistic? Yes, but surely a brutal society starts by brutalising its children.

Give me the posters that tell of action for children's welfare, happiness and freedom and the autonomous struggle that starts in anger and ends in a party.

## LEARNING COURAGE FROM MY STEPMOTHER

This stern face,
Sternly turns towards me,
I cower

### John Hoggett

And observe the kitchen lino.
It has large black and white squares,
Well used, scratched, but still serviceable,
In need of a sweep too.

For fifteen years
This stern face
Sternly turned towards me.
From age ten to twenty five,
I cowered
And studied the kitchen lino.
But no more.
One day, while she while she went to work
I packed a small bag,
Chequebook and switch card at the bottom,
Wrapped in my pyjamas.
And walked out.

I see her occasionally,
Out of the corner of my eye,
In Sainsbury's or the library.
I blink and she is gone.
She blinks her eye and I'm not there,
In Sainsbury's, the library of the park,
I am gone.

People face me sternly.
I stare at the floor,
Then say, 'Tut tut, such bad manners,'
Or laugh and laugh and laugh,
Get out my mirror and say,
'Do you want to see your face?'

# FIRST BOOK

'Let me show you your face.'
And laugh and laugh and laugh.


## DIVINITY

I,
Am God.
Which may,
Explain why,
Your life is so strange.


## PERSONAL CONSTRUCT THEORY

We trade in images, you and I.
I give you a 1964 Batman bubblegum card,
You give me a pebble you found on some beach.
For you it shone like the moon under romance.
For me it fits in with the gravel on the drive.
We shared a joke over the Batman card,
It showed someone dressed like a mutual friend of
ours.
We trade in images you and I
And sometimes that trade is uneven,
Though politeness, thank God, stops us from
saying so.

## UNTITLED 7

In Alcoholics Anonymous they have various bits of street wisdom like, 'STOP,' 'THINK,' and, 'DON'T BE SUCH A GIT!' They also say that living with an alcoholic is like living with an elephant in the living room where no one is allowed to mention it.

To which I have added that, if you do mention it then you risk seeing a family member become so upset that you wonder if they are going to have a nervous breakdown, being made homeless, losing that family inheritance, suffering violence, or what is perhaps worse for some of us, the humiliation of being laughed at.

For me, thinking about, talking about, and acting on, the inescapability of global warming, the thinning of the ozone layer and massive global pollution is in some ways similar.

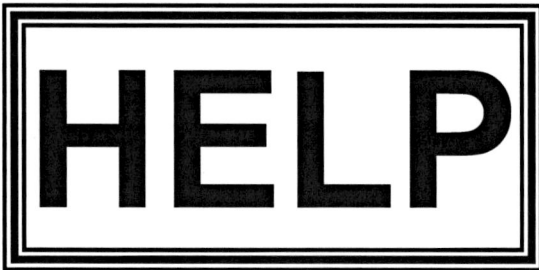

# HELP

# FIRST BOOK

## UNTITLED 8

Twenty years ago I first started learning abut global pollution. Today, the 1$^{st}$ of February 1995, we have floods all over Europe. I am tempted to glow with that smug glib happiness as I rush around saying, 'I told you so'.

## SICKNESS

He said, 'It's influenza,' I said, 'It's only a cold.'
He said, 'I'm sick as a dog.' I said, 'You're not even in a sweat.'
He said, 'Fold me in your arms.' I said, 'We've only just met.'

## REMINDER TO MYSELF

I've got M.E., a tummy bug, and when that isn't tiring me out and filling my time, flashbacks.

What do I want a revolution for? I want a revolution where when I'm ill, a friend comes round to ask how I am, do the shopping and cook me dinner instead of saying, 'Maybe.' When I ask him round and I'm ill, he's got a week off work, isn't going anywhere and lives three doors down the road. Where I don't come third best to getting stoned, watching Neighbours, and on a good night, playing computer games.

What's wrong with me? I choose cruddy friends, that's what, and I'm bitter as hell about it. Just leave 'em to rot in their hell-holes of alcohol and drug abuse and the social actions of frightened three-year olds (you stole my Dinky car so I'm gonna sit in my room and whine).

They've got as much understanding and sympathy as my mother, drunk or hung over the next day.

None – zilch – zero, and dangerous with it, well they are to my 21$^{st}$ century damaged psyche (or should that read pride?)

Fuck 'em, it's sad, and they are: lonely insecure straight men, who either don't have girlfriends and agonise over it, or psuedo, posy, bullies, who rant at their girlfriends in the street. Oh save me, I've got better things to do.

Where are the people that care? 'Cause I'm on the look out for them.

Time was when I was on holiday at Gay Men's Week (new age, hippy, slightly socialist, but oh so groovy gay Men's Week, mainstay of my sanity for the last five years) when this guy got ill with a really bad gut ache. Finally he/we wanted to take him to hospital; not only was a driver found but he was asked who, from amidst a crowd of almost complete stranger, he would like to accompany him on the ride.

He was amazed, I thought, 'Well isn't that normal?' Well not round here – no. Here you'll get ignored for two weeks, then someone will come round to ask for that record they lent you three weeks ago, and when you say you were too ill, they say, 'Oh yeah – never mind' – and walk out, like you need forgiveness for not returning a record when you're so ill you can hardly go down the corner shop.

If this goes on much longer I'll start throwing things – honest I will.

At least with queens you know when you've fallen out by the dirty looks, and they say, 'I've been telling all my friends about what you did,' not that you know what you did, but hey! Then you don't speak to each other for six months – three years, whatever – but you knew that before you did fall out you had what might reasonable be called a friendship where you had dinner together, told jokes at each other's expense, but if you went too far and hurt each other's feelings you said so and talked about it. You cried on each other's shoulders at opportune and inopportune moments and you flirted in the break in the Betty Davies movie on TV. Then, if needed, you had an in-depth discussion of whether this was a serious flirtation with invite to bed thrown in, a bit of fun

*John Hoggett*

over the home made popcorn, or was this some kind of confused horror trip that no self respecting queen got herself into and can we sort this out. Now! Please! Hey, maybe that's where we fell out? But at least you knew it was a friendship.

And where, I hear you ask, are the women? Well honey, what with mother dying when I was nine, being touched up by my sister when I was ten and Dad marrying one of his less attractive students later that year (she was an alcoholic, or went that way after living with Dad for a while, and if treated her the way the straight men I know treat me, Honey I can understand) I guess women are not my first port of call in a storm.

So for me, all women really are potential drunks or perverts, until proved otherwise. And if that isn't 'Right on,' then tough. I support Women's Aid, Rape Crises, equal opportunities for women, good child care facilities and one hundred other things on the feminist agenda.

'All Men Are Rapists,' went the 80's feminist slogan and I know what drove them to anti-male hate-ridden sloganising. I know about the levels of violence in the home, on the street, wherever; the harassment women get from men at work; the intimidation that is reinforced by the media that always shows frightened women suffering rape and assault and never, ever shows self respecting women fighting back, and mocks any self respecting women fighting back; and mocks any self directed movement by women (vis Reclaim The Night marches, not loved by our Tory Tabloid press, but then all victors mock the attempts of the vanquished to fight back, it is the first tool of power, throw a few names and make a fool of 'em, see if that'll keep 'em quiet). Or trivialising them like straight men turning Riot Girrrls into figures of lust – oh please, spare me from it, you miss the point with almost deliberate dull-wittedness.

But now I'm stating how I feel, this deep lack of trust, of everyone I suppose, women included. It's a personal thing, how I've been brought up. And don't talk to me about professionals, my parents were social workers.

I don't' want no part in any struggle that doesn't honour how I feel.

And if you say, 'Aren't you being a little bitter?' 'Taking this a little too seriously/personally?' 'Digging up the past?' 'Over-dramatising a little?' 'Being a fucked up little Drama Queen.' 'Wanting more than most people have to give, maybe you just need to accept things the way they are?' 'Maybe it was meant to be like this?' Or the New Age-ier than thou, 'What have you got to learn from this, John?' I'll say, 'Why don't you fuck off and come back when you're wearing something more interesting – like that little lurex and diamante number perhaps?'

Well that's me for tonight – ciao baby ciao – and lets hope they sort out my sickness benefit claim soon so I can get a much needed taxi to the shoperama. I'm here, I'm queer and I'm gonna buy me something special, black olives, smoked German cheese and a "God Is My Co-Pilot" album, if Mark Connorton raves about them so much they must have something that'll make my pecker rise.


## THE MOODY THERAPIST

The Moody Therapist will help you feel,
      Guide you to see;
That you are a child of the Sun,
      That the Moon shines down on you,
      That the Earth sees you as one of her more
beautiful                   flowers.

The Moody Therapist will go home
To a life of scowling houses,
Washing up not done:
Ancient resentments, piled up.
      Psychic muck encrusted in the kitchen,
      House-mates scattering to their rooms.
The Moody Therapist sees himself
      As talented but suffering,
Others are of divided opinions,
But some perhaps are his friends.

# FIRST BOOK

---

There are more strange people in the world than there are people.

---

## WHINGERS

They show me their bleeding-heart,
Cut their wrist poetry;
And I say, "Oh sod off,"
"Give us a cup of tea - grow up, go away,"
"Get a life and leave me alone,"
"I'm off."

Off on me bike:
I cycle for miles,
Through country lanes lined with trees;
Behind men on tractors,
Stopped by cows at milking time, waddling,
In the lanes, between field and farm.
Then on, cycling on to nowhere,
Filled with hedge lined views.

Home is where the whingers are;
Suffer little whingers, suffer.
I'll sit and sew and think of them.
Then do the washing up,
Listen to Radio Four;
More whingers on the radio,
Oh Hell!

*John Hoggett*

Joe Grundy, Linda Snell, World at one, Poetry
Now.
I'll put a record on instead;
Bloody Neil Young, the Blues, Janice Joplin.
Home is where the whingers are - oh yeah:
Slit your wrist, go on.
I'll come to your funeral,
Dance on whinger, party on.


## THE STRANGER AT THE DOOR

The stranger at the door,
No one asked him,
He brings no gift.

Does he smile,
Does he not?
Shall I ask Him?
Shall I not?
Do I owe him?
Do I not?
Is he stone,
Is he not?
Is he friend;
Potential,
Remembered,
Unknown,
Lost but not found again;
Is he not?

The stranger at the door,

# FIRST BOOK

What is he to me?
Where am I for him?

Would I be a Stranger at someone's door?
The frozen knock,
Standing, not moving, a question not formed.
Ah - the stranger at the door.


## BY THE RISING OF THE SUN

Some people are no longer speaking to me.
Their silence says more than all they previously
had to say.
Eyes are averted when I enter the room,
Coffee cups are studiously studied:
Thus I know I have significance in their life,
And all is well with the world.


## SILLY LITTLE BITTER OLD QUEEN

Mike - 19 - Handsome - 19 any age.
Cheeks like a teddy bear,
Naturally rouged.
Did he revisit Brideshead?

A girlfriend called Kalie,
Goddess of love, Goddess of destruction.
At home, when younger he lived opposite a
woman, old,

Husband dead, she spent her time sewing, and
making rag rugs,
She had many.
I make rag rugs, a hobby.
He asked me if I would make one for him,
"Make one for me, big enough for my bed,"
Warm, comfortable, cosy.
I said, "No, it would take too long."
Mike - 19 - Handsome - 19 any age.
Girlfriend called Kalie,
Goddess of love, Goddess of destruction.

A  rug of rags.

Love,
Possession,
Love.

A cosy bundle of love,
Not mine.

Years ago I would have written long, passionate
letters,
Not posted them, pined.
Maybe sat on doorsteps, drank a solitary bottle of
wine,
Said embarrassing things and not remembered
them.
Years later I would have got the letters out and
tortured myself with them.
Now, I write poems and read them out for our
mutual embarrassment.

## THE BEAUTY OF GAY MEN

The beauty of Gay Men eluded me for years;
But now I see it in shop doors,
Pubs, clubs, cafes and bus shelters.
They smile; warm, knowingly,
Inviting or just acknowledging, enjoying the view.
I am beautiful, a gay man, my beauty is
The beauty of the homosexual - love.  Here today,
gone today; here again soon.
Beauty, love, Beauty.

## IN THE PHOENIX GARDENS BEHIND ST GILES IN THE FIELDS CHURCH

Gay men sit on benches, holding hands, talking of
intimacy.
A child plays in the pile of grass cuttings.
A lesbian cuts the grass, leaving neat lines:
Such a summer, Sunday-afternoon sound, that
word;
Lesbians.
Lazy, lounging, lesbians watch,
While their friend mows the lawn.
In the Phoenix Gardens just behind
          St Giles in the fields church.

# RULE - DO THE MOST IMPORTANT THINGS LAST

I seem to have a rule in my head that goes, "Leave the most important things 'til last."

I wonder if we will treat our world's environmental problems in the same way?
I myself, usually, despite the panic and self hatred, manage to get my projects in, completed, finished. Maybe not with the total polish of a truly modern professional, but with a certain panache, humanness and room to breath. But will the Human Race?
After all, many of us consistently fail, make a huge mess of our lives, leave things till far too late and live uncomfortable, desperate lives with uncompromisingly stupid beliefs in slogan's like, 'This time it'll be all right,' 'The love of a 'Good man',' 'If he/she/God really loved me (with the resultant disappointment ten minutes, one hour, one day, ten years later when you find out he/she/God doesn't really know what either you or love is and is far too busy mending his Mechano set (God), saving the world from evil through prayer and a new accounting system (men) or .......... (well I never was too good on women anyway.......).

# FIRST BOOK

## CHANGING THE RULES

Changing the rules of the game:
From football to billiards, billiards to net-ball;
Tiddlywinks or tiger hunting, on the backs of an elephant.
"Ere, what's your game?"
"Are you a playmate?"
Is this the game of the month, match of the day, or a lifegame?
If I am one up, how do I know if you are down far enough?
Do I need patience or should I snap?
The crack of willow on leather, the cracking of heads:
"All's fair in love and war"; and the playing fields of Eton are not far from here.
Some games are "non-competitive", they don't seem very popular after the age of five.
The farmer's in his den, we all pat the dog;
He collapses to the playground floor, grazing his knees;
We pile on top, he screams, we laugh and more pile on.
Changing the rules of the game,
I wouldn't know where to start.
The referee's out, the umpire's bored to death,
But the scoreboard still stands steady.
Changing the rules of the game,
I don't know where to begin.
"Well, shall we start from here then?"
"Let's start at the very beginning,"

"ABC, Doe Ray Mee," ready steady,
On your marks, get set;
I don't know where to begin.
Changing the rules of the game,
I wouldn't know were to start.
Changing the rules of the game,
I don't know where to begin.


## CURRICULUM VITAE

Curriculum vitae,
Let me sleep and say,
Nothing.
Rumour and dissonance,
Power and merrydance,
Knitting.
Work, it's a pile of shit,
Friends a load of gits,
Fucking.

Farmers
Pollute the world;
Fertilise and aphidcide,
Spray the veg,
Spray the men,
Take it home,
Start again.

Curriculum vitae,
Let me sleep and say,
Nothing.

# FIRST BOOK

Rumour and dissonance,
Power and merrydance,
Knitting.
Work, it's a pile of shit,
Friends a load of gits,
Fucking.


## MATTHEW

Matthew, Matty, Mr Shenstone:
Moody git, moody bastard, sick.
So sick, so moody, we ran away.
Sorry matey, Matty, Matt;
Gone away, dead, gone, bye.
Funeral missed - contact lost, tara.


## TARA

Tara Matey - Johny, John.
Gone to Heaven where dogs roam free.
They come here, home, home to me.
Moody, they don't care,
They come to me.
Tara matey, in my heaven me.

*John Hoggett*

## STONE

'Write a poem for me,' she said, 'go on.'

No I won't, no I won't, no I won't.

I'll write it with a broken biro, smeared:
Smudged with finger prints, black.
I'll sit here in this chair,
You won't see me, ugly;
Ugly as you, ugly as you, ugly as you.

## THEOLOGY

If we create God in our own image, or as the
Greek philosopher Xenophanes commented, the
Ethiopians have black, snub nosed Gods while the
Thracians have blue eyed, red haired ones, then
my God will be polite, have a hankering for tea
and make scones on an irregular, though not
infrequent basis.

## THE CREED

If we have such concepts as a 'Holy War' or 'Jihad'
or 'Just War' why can we not have a 'Holy
Friendship,' a divine embroidering of a holy prayer
shawl, or recognise that the road to heaven can
be most quickly consecrated by the holding of

hands by friends in the kitchen, the market place
or in the fields.


## CENSOR

I censor myself for you.
I censor myself for you.
I censor myself to protect you.

Lies lies lies.

I censor myself for me.
I censor myself - careful.
I censor myself to protect me -danger.

The phone - you and me - silence.
Held - holding the phone - miles in between:
Silence.
Not saying, not thinking.
The wall, the silence.
Censor.


## PHILOSOPHY

I've been miserable for years,
It's a career I have.
It doesn't pay the rent,
And it's not part of Labour's New Deal;
But it keeps me off the streets at night,

Brooding,
Inconsolable,
Lonely.
You see it's all my fault;
The deaths
The break downs (friends, family, lovers),
The betrayals (I've specialised, mainly, in unfaithful men).
So you see,
It's all my fault,
I'm dangerous to people,
Not that I'm vain, I hope you don't misunderstand me,
But I am dangerous.
It's true.
So keep well away,
I do - I keep myself to myself.
It's a career I have,
For safety - yours and mine.
It has its compensations and I've been miserable for years,
I keep off the streets at night.

Take care.

---

Nobody loves me very much, just a little bit, on Tuesday afternoons.

---

# FIRST BOOK

## UNGENDERING

Ed said, that I make him camp.
Standing next to me his bones go fluffy:
Head lisps to one side, lips pout,
Hair reeks of unmanageability.
It's all my fault, says Ed;
Denying, absolutely, all responsibility.
And him with a girlfriend too.

## REPULSIVE MAGNETS

I walk around in a cloud
Of taciturn, moody, pushawayness,
That says, 'Piss off, go away, bog off'

They come near, smile,
Say how much they like my work
My performance,
Me.

How perverse.

## MY FAVOURITE CV

Newbury was my flowering, it was where I shone:
Battles with busses, stopping security guards
going to work;
Street stalls and shouting;
Collecting money from noisy bars at chucking out
time;
Meetings where everyone listened - no one
yawned and 20 decisions were made by
consensus in 1 1/2 hours;
Arguments over 'tree spiking' and the sanctity of
workers      verses the sanctity of the trees;
Visiting prisoners, supporting prison visitors with
tea and talk;
 Putting on gigs, performing on stage,
Hiring PA's, halls, lighting rigs and god knows
what else,
Working with Prima Donna's, committed hippies,
stars, lovers of the land and friends;
Cooking for weekend protesters, collecting wood
for tree       houses;
Going with Marie to buy her first ever climbing
harness;
Building 'lock-on's' at Snelsmore;
Building a water store for a garden there, too;
Flirting outrageously and finally getting, or should
that be sharing, a shag?
Training in Non violent Direct Action (history
lessons on the       Suffragettes, Ghandi, Mothers
of The Disappeared,        Greenham, CND);

# FIRST BOOK

Training in Stress Management and Community
Building;
Then later on, training on court procedure and
learning from our mistakes;
Making press releases, then being on the radio,
on TV, in the press;
Making phone trees, making 3am phone calls;
Standing around, watching friends be evicted from
trees,
Feeling cold, useless and angry,
Swearing, "I'll never do that again,"
Going home, learning form it, resting, resting and
resting,
Coming back better prepared, hopefully;
Arguments with work colleagues, discussions with
friends;
Talking in pubs after meetings, having socials,
parties, video evenings, food;
Deciding what to spend our funds on (rope and
tilley lamps for Snelsmore's Gotan camp);
All of us using our lifetime's experience on this,
And from it we got a lifetime's worth of experience.
Newbury was our flowering, it was where we
shone.

*John Hoggett*

## THE WAY OF IT ALL

I love that nice guy, nasty guy routine,
Love me, hate me
Slap me, smile.
Kiss me, bite a bit,
Trash my room then cook my favourite lunch.

I'm putty in your hands my love,
I'm putty in your hands.

I love that nice guy, nasty guy routine;
I'm stern, and scowl, though like to think I'm fair,
I'm firm, but proud, in the gentleness of the air.
Don't cross this line and it'll be fine,
We can dance and we can eat,
Do the Fandango, eat chocolate and
Parade about in the street.
Behind the prickly hedge is our garden, so divine.


## THIS IS A SAD HOME FOR SAD BOYS

This is a Sad Home for Sad Boys,
This is a Sad Home for Sad Boys,
Ashley said.
This is a Sad Home for Sad Boys.
This is a dress rehearsal for a drama school for
another life.
My life will begin when I am fifty five,
When I will be reborn as a teenager;
Wise and lively, excited all the time, full of friends.

# FIRST BOOK

This is a Sad Home for Sad Boys.

Our friend is not suicidal,
Our friend is not suicidal,
Our friend is not suicidal.
We know no-body.
We don't know anybody who eats ninety pounds
worth of heroin for breakfast,
And cries because he pukes it up - not dead.
This is a Sad Home for Sad Boys.

This house is a sad house where sad boys live,
We know of no acquaintances that have died of
heroin.
We know no-one.
No-one who was angry, hurt and disabled.
No-one, angry, very hurt and scary.
No-one scary.
We know of no-one who died of heroin.

We know no-one,
We are not scared,
This is a sad house for sad boys.
The music is ugly and blares,
No one cares.
The music is ugly and blares,
No one cares.
The music is ugly and blares,
No one cares.

Our friends do not steal our money,
Our friends do not tell us they know best.,

*John Hoggett*

Our friends do not tell us lies.
We have no friends.
This is a Sad Home for Sad Boys.

There are no links between heroin, death and the
economy.
Society does not exist, it is a figment of a non-
imagination.
I will bow my head then drink my beer.
A man asked,
"Why do you think it is your responsibility?"
I do not.
I have no friends.
This is a Sad Home for Sad Boys.

My friend says, "Why do you seethe?  You enjoy
it, don't you."
I do not, it is what I do.
I swim in the sea of impossibilities.
I have no friends.

I need to talk to no-one.
I have no problems.
My friends tell me what to do.
This is a Sad Home for Sad Boys.
This is where the sad boys live.
Ashley said.

# FIRST BOOK

## TOTALLY UNREAL DADDY

Daddy - a walk by the river (when we are five).

Daddy - a "hey that's interesting" when I tell him I'm gay, and years later he welcomes the new boyfriend into his house.

Daddy admires my bike and the way I ride it. Helps with the difficult jobs like adjusting the brake blocks.

Daddy - loves mum and lets me know it.

Daddy - mum dies, I am eight years old. Daddy stays at home from work for two weeks, Sis and me stay home from school. He goes through mum's clothes and belongings with us deciding what to throw out and what to keep, stopping to see how we are, explaining our questions, giving us little mementos of her, putting others by for when we are older; introducing us gently to the idea of the funeral. He is slow, considerate, taking care of himself while caring of us. Love flows between us in these grief filled moments.

Daddy - so interested in me that sometimes, when I go to see him, I have to sit him down and give him a cup of tea before telling him how work / love / home, is for me at the moment.

Daddy - telling me about how, in Germany after the war, he had wondered if he himself was Gay, tells me how he sees men now - interesting - we share our views; in many ways similar, in many more ways different; mine developed in the years since I made that decision, age 17, that gay is easier, makes more sense, is comfort and comfortable for me. Years of boyfriends, lovers, flirting, sex, lust, breaking up and making up, heartache and healing, hate, miserableness and high-kicking, deep-sighing, love: his from a different life, different.

We talk of women, a little; we share some details of how we see women, a little, just a little, then stop. We think of the women in his life, of our different relationships to them, and stop, reflect, talk of something else.

Daddy - there to tell us (I was nine years old, my sister thirteen), me and Sis, that he is ready to remarry; to ask us, and to listen to more than our words, to spend time on how we feel about this. We are young - children -young.

Daddy - sensing our feeling about our potential step-mother, sits down and thinks, then talks it over with us; talks it over with her; considers, brings us together as a family / potential family - we talk, we discuss, we fight and argue and struggle and live with each other, each taking time, over the years, to get to know each other - Daddy.

Daddy - his wife, my steomother, leaving him, I am twenty. He stops, apologises, we share a look that says, "I am sorry". Daddy - broken, sharing my brokenness; I, sharing his. I grow up a little - Daddy - his pain is great, mine is too.

Daddy - he recovers, slowly, and remarries, his third wife. I am welcomed into the home, get to know his new wife; he is tentative, concerned about how his children and his new wife get on,

knowing both are, to him, important, and knowing both to be adults; his wisdom stretched on how to deal with this delicate situation, but he tries.
Daddy.
Daddy - sensing his children growing up , becoming independent, watches their mistakes and triumphs, - welcomes their visits and remembers his children's favourite food on their birthdays.
Daddy, tries to make a home for them in their new home with his now, not so new wife.
Daddy.
But this Daddy is one I have created out of fantasy and hazy-half memories to be put away in the freezer and pulled out and defrosted when I need him; when times are hard and when times are good and I need someone to tell it to - Daddy - mine. I made him, he is part of me - my creation.
Daddy.

*John Hoggett*

## THE QUEER CHILD

The Queer Child, a boy, collects buttons, sews daises on blankets, and wistfully follows footballers, but with no eye for the game. He plays tag, dislikes getting his fingers muddy but watches those that play with mud from a distance. On his Christmas list are washing machines and vacuum cleaners, kitchen cupboard, mincers, food processors; the sharpening of carving knives fascinate him as much as, or more than, tractors, diggers and cars. He knows his role, grows into it happily, those around him know it too, and despite their embarrassment and mild disapproval they know the Queer boy will grow to be the Queer Man who will bring his Queer tales to their hearth. Despite their pretence and protestation they look forward to this. Their pretence and protestation is only for the neighbours sake after all.

## SINGLE PARENTHOOD

Alone, lonely, again.
The dark, lonely cave
Where the solitary child
Sits, and anxiously waits.
Scurrying into his bedtime blankets
Before Daddy sneaks in,
Angry that his children demand his attention.
His evening of simple high living spoiled
By the complexity of parenting.
A task that eludes this high living Dad;
It slips through his fingers.
He is both careless of , and irritated by,
The loneliness and desolation of his children.
The children play and bicker,
Riding from mania to cruelty,
In that journey peculiar to neglected children.

*John Hoggett*

# THE AGE OF UNREASON

I like to fuck
And suck
And cluck
Tut tut, dear me, well I never,
They didn't do that in my day.

Well of course we did,
But quietly,
With Dignity,
Style,
Panache,
And Mother certainly never knew.

And if she did it too
Well that was that.
It was certainly never mentioned over tea.
Not in our house anyway.
Neither should it be,
And I hope you're the same.
So off you go to bed now,
And I'll hear no more of that sort of talk out of you.
So run along now.
And goodnight,
Seep well, goodnight.

# FIRST BOOK

## I AM MY OWN HERO

I am my own hero.
I can be seen
In the green room of Radio Four chat shows.
Peter Purves phones me when he is feeling down.
I have never met John Noakes
But we took his dog for a walk
When the dog handler was sick.
Carter the Unstoppable Sex Machine
Use me for their backing singer.
They say they would much rather
Use someone they know and like
Rather than one of those professionals form the agency,
And sometimes I help Fruitbat programme his drum machine.
Just on the song he wrote about me,
Well partly about me - you know the one?
Diana wrote to me once.
But I like to keep the Royals at a distance,
Not get involved.
It would spoil the fun of seeing how they run.
Little Royal piggies running this way and that.
Whereas if I get involved I would have to have a serious opinion,
Be friends with some, enemies with others.
So I wrote back.
Actually I got my personal assistant to do it.
I've got standards you know.
As I often say,
"You've got to put yourself first,"

And I am my own hero.


## EXORCISM FOR HIM

Cast out this Heterosexual Demon!
Make him gay
As he should be.
Cast out this Demon of Darkness,
This false deflowerer of this elegant youth.
Let his true nature shine forth,
His young manly body lying with a young manly body,
Their sweat intermingles as they share this family bed.
Let love fly into and through him
And bring forth the proper flowering of love
Once more into this house.


## THE BISEXUAL FILES

Having a Bisexual Boyfriend means not knowing whom he fancies more, Scully or Mulder.
Having a Bisexual Boyfriend means not knowing whether he fancies Scully or Mulder or both of them, and if both of them, which one does he prefer tonight? Or is it both of them, together, at once, in one bed, in one fantasy, in one imagination, and that's his.
Having a Bisexual Boyfriend can be mysterious, sometimes it can be a little confusing and leave

you feeling you've been left in the dark. From time to time you may feel theirs is an alien world just around the corner, just out of reach. And are these aliens; friends or foe? And do they want to find you?

Having a Bisexual boyfriend opens up a whole new world of possibility, and in all probability, one you'll never know. One he lives in and on some level that world will always remain strange to you. He inhabits that world and in all probability he will always be a puzzle to you.

## ROUND HERE THE MEN HUG EACH OTHER

Round here the men hug each other:
On greeting after long partings,
      the reuniting of old friends;
On greeting after returning from the shops,
      the reuniting over the sorting of groceries;
On waking up, on going to bed;
In joy shared, in comfort and despair,
With sexual thrill and without,
On completing an essay,
On the occasion of mutual forgiveness
For wrongs both slight and intractable,
While walking down the street,
While walking cliff tops, sand dunes, tree lined lanes,
In the foyer of motor-way service stations;
As acts of protest,
As acts of ease;

In imagination, in actuality,
On paper and through the post;
As acts of compassion, admiration and flirtation;
It is a language that knows no rhyme and no reason,
It is a language that knows no rhyme and infinite reason;
All I know is that men hug each other
Round here.


## I WANT TO BE MISERABLE FOREVER

I want to be miserable forever.
I want to pout and pine, unrepentantly, amongst unsympathetic friends,
And live in rented houses which leak, where landlords try half-heartedly to evict me at intermittent and unpredictable times.
I want to be successful in my endeavours every seven months,
Not try again for another six years,
And think, "Well, it's not what I really want to do."
I want my friends and lovers to die and I want to never quite get over it;
To grieve when my other friends are partying and vice versa.
I want to join a union, because the principle is good, the history fantastic and my managers and management committee are manipulative bitches and ineffective men (though all in rather low-level, pathetic ways).

# FIRST BOOK

I want to join a union where the people are such that I would rather sit in my room and re-read a page from The Guardian twenty times than talk to them.

I want to join a new-age, therapeutic movement which wants to "Save the World," where ninety-five percent of it's members are from the educated middle classes, for whom thousands of years of politics and history are unfortunate, and the ugly facts of life are best not discussed.

I want to realise that my love life has been horrible and ugh for 20 years,

Find weekend courses where I can learn something about this, knowing that one weekend is the educational equivalent of the registration day for a university course, and I am surrounded by people desperate to see me unchanged.

I want to discover the horrors of my childhood:

Make useful comparisons to survivors of war,

Then worry about forgiving the bastards/confronting the bastards for the next 15, 20, 300 years.

I want to protest against the building of the Newbury Bypass, see it built, protest some more, this time about the resulting in-fill development, heavy-metal run-off, global warming; hear about massive international pollution in Italy, Spain, Thailand, Borneo, Georgia and the Unfortunately United States of America.

Write to my MP, (a sleazy geezer I've known for 15 years),

Set fire to myself on the steps of St Paul's,

Join small protest groups with people who make
me cringe,
Or go to bed for a few weeks, months, years.
I want to be miserable for years.
At last I have a realisable ambition.


## TO TOUCH THE MOON

We made love once, him and I,
Shall I tell you what it was like, shall I?

Was it like, was it like
Horses, pounding on a tide swept beach,
Hooves, sending up storm swept spray?
Was it, was it?
Maybe,
But then again.

Was it like, was it like
Flowers, caressed by a late spring, summer sun,
Opening to receive it's warming rays?
Perhaps, Maybe,
But, well, then again.

Well was it, was it,
Was it like, fish, swimming around green, cool,
river weed,
On a sultry, hot, summers day.
Perhaps, sort of,
I'm not sure.

# FIRST BOOK

But afterwards,
We thoughtfully, thoughtlessly slept;
And in the morning
He went downstairs to fetch cereal, fruit, coffee
and the papers,
While I curled up around the warm memory
Of something
I had somehow
Forgotten
To remember.


## PERSONAL GROWTH MANTRA

They say that I will grow
They say that I will grow
They say that I will grow

People shrink when they get older.


## WHITE PUNKS IN DRAG

I'm a fucked up queen and I don't care,
I paint my nails and dye my hair,
I go out with men I don't like,
They fuck me up but that's all right.

## REPETITION COMPLEX

Practising conversations in my head,
Practising conversations in my head,
Practising conversations in my head;
Oh God, I'd rather watch TV.

## SEX POSITIVE

I had sex and it was fun,
Tiddly-dum, Tiddly-dum, Tiddly-dum.

## TO ALL THE GAY FOOTBALLERS

Knickers,
Knackers.
Knobs,
Cor!

## Homo Sensuality

Some like it on the tum,
I like it up the bum.

## DIVINITY II

I am god
Which is all right by me.

# FIRST BOOK

## SANCTUARY

I sit in my room,
Stare at the floor;
Sanctuaries are quiet places.


## MABEL'S RAGE
## OR
## MARRIAGE AND INCONVENIENCE

To all you unfaithful men,
Grow up!


## DINNER WITH THE LITERATI

I know the stories that reel the fishes in,
Rich fish, rich fish,
Dinners coming in.


## CON

Con,
Got a gob on, Con.
Plays harmonica, Con.
Wish he'd play harmonica all day long.
That'd stop the gob that Con's got on.

## FASHION VERSES TRENDINESS

"It's trendy to be bisexual" - something that is constantly said about young bisexuals, especially men.

Well I think it's true. I personally have gone beyond trendy and am now inhabiting the outer reaches of wacky - like one of those cheeses that have been left hanging around too long and look, interesting, with 'approach with care' written on them.

But there must be so called straight men who must ache to be trendier. Their clothes, hair, papers they read, TV programmes they watch, videos they rent just don't say "Trendy" - just vaguely interesting. Even the way they walk could be construed as bordering on the boring. Well perhaps a little flirtation with bisexuality might make them very trendy indeed.

I mean, look at Michael Portillo. Actually, don't look at Michael Portillo, I'd rather you didn't. Instead, look at his friend, Ivan Massow; gay man, personal finance expert for the gay community, millionaire, potential candidate for the Mayor of London - a very good person to see if you want to talk pensions, not so good if you want to talk politics and policies. Personally, I think Red Ken as the Mayor of London would be better for the Lesbian, Gay and Bisexual Community; at least for the community I want to support. But Mr Portillo came out of the closet, while reaffirming his present heterosexual state, long enough before any general election for any furore to die down but using it to get his name in the press, get his political ambitions recognised, link his name to Mr Hague (in a non sexual way of course) and springboard his rather flagging career. And all without ever mentioning his policies! How clever, the epitome of "Trendy".

Now there must be some heterosexual chap out there who feels his image is less than interesting? Would any of you like to be trendy? I am available for an interesting assignation and I'm sure many of my friends could provide the gossip - thus boosting your importance and indeed your trendiness in one simple night of pleasure, go on, treat yourself – be trendy!


## THE POEM OF PRAYERS


With beech trees and pressed leaves,
With cool streams and bath-toy boats,
With fresh and pressed grasses,
With garlic-mustard and summer dust,
With dew dropped lettuce and ice shattered cabbage,
With cold shattered hands and mustard hot sandwich,

*John Hoggett*

With this that and the other,
A goodbye-good morning wave from mother,
And the thousand mile walk from the garden gate
 To       the       weight       of       a       lover,
From the Dawn of the World to the death of our
Dad,
From spinning top silver twirl to the finger chewed
slinky girl,
From Silverkrin images to Anarchist riot,
From storeyville hometown to city slick bar-b-que,
From sex confused easy boy to blown away easy
toy,
The World turns every day 'cause life says it is
that way,
We pray for the rain knowing it will come someday
anyway,
I pray for the rain knowing rain and the cold and
the refreshing and the hurricane,
I pray for the rain knowing prayers and the pain,
I pray.

# FIRST BOOK

## THE END OF THE WORLD AS WE KNOW IT

*(Y2K and all that)*

"It's the end of the world" said Paul,
"Trains will jam up as the signals fail,
Cities will jam up as the traffic lights fail,
The electricity will end, gas supplies stop,
Water will stop flowing from the tap and the sewers will overflow,
The banks will forget how much money they hold,
There will be no housing benefit, job seekers allowance or disability        allowance,
Nuclear industries will become like sieves, the uranium and plutonium will flow out where once it trickled,
The radio, TV, telephone and newspapers will all stop,
The shops will run out of food,
There will be disease, illness and cold.
"The World ends everyday," said John,
"In the betrayal of friends, family and lovers,
The destruction of the ozone layer by chemicals manufactured to power freezers,
The catastrophic destruction of the rainforest for the production of junk mail,
The death of young men way before their time,
The everyday rape of children by adults and older siblings,
It's just the end of the world," said John,
"It's just the end of the world".

**TAKING IT EASY**
**or**
**THE BLACK SHEEP**

I will become the Bishop of Ease
And end my days as the Monk of Sloth.
My love life will consist of eyeing, round corners,
Handsome young men, who, for perversities sake,
We shall, inaccurately, call boys,
And shall spy them on wet Wednesday
afternoons, in April, November and January.
My body will have the casual mis-shapeliness
Of those whose diet consists of Waitrose
Chocolate Swiss-Roll,
Occasionally topped with evaporated milk
To comfort against the loss of not very favourite
jumpers.

I will write poems one month, the next, in two,
three, five, eight
And fourteen month intervals
In broken approximation to some mathematician's
delight.
My achievements will be celebrated
By afternoons spent in bed - alone,
Sometimes dressed in flannelette pyjamas
And just occasionally, just to feel the contrast, in
none.

Someday, someone may try to give me an
honorary degree
For filling in that most bureaucratic of fictions,

# FIRST BOOK

My "Record Of Jobs Applied For" form in record
quick time,
But I shall turn it down, not welcoming the fame or
approbation.
And one day, it being Sunday,
I will invite a solitary friend and his pal,
Who has been known to go hill walking near
Aylesbury,
Round for tea
To celebrate twenty-one years of uninterrupted
signing on.

Some speak of a walk through life,
Others have a carefully worked out plan
Stuck to with rigidity and determinism
I will merely snooze through mine.
And any nightmare I see in the distance
Will signal a detour through the valleys
Or a short/long stop at a stone-built cosy tea
house
For hours, days, months or years if necessary.
"Oh well," will be one of my favourite phrases,
And, "Whatever," my reply to any question that
I deem at all difficult - and that will probably be
most of them.

My life will be a bed of ease, not sleaze;
A slightly grubby, very untidy one, with a few
crumbs perhaps.
And hey, Tuesday is my favourite day of the week
And this is just a poem.
So.................

## ROUGH LOVE

He squeezed him until he spat out the pip,
Squashed oranges, baked potatoes, carrots.
Neither realised that this love affair was over.

## TERROR NIGHTS

Repulsive;
Ugly life of rock,
Lie still,
Recall those misfits
And scream.

---

Suddenly I was lost in my own flat.  Someone had
dropped some acid in the mushroom bhaji.

---

## REMEMBRANCE OF TIMES PAST

*Lord forgive me for I have stolen someone else's title.*

The time was we would enter strange houses,
Smoke strong drugs with strangers;
Time would collapse,
Expand again
And we would suffer no harm.

# FIRST BOOK

Time was we would skip down the street
Hand in Hand,
Occasionally whinnying like horses,
Stopping at out of the way post offices
To cash our giros.

Time was
Time was

Time was we would throw wild parties
And "sleep" with our best friend and his lover
On a coat covered floor
With the other party guests crowded around us,
Then involuntarily cry out loudly as we came;
Our party guests laughing in embarrassed delight
at our crowing.

Time was

Time was we would visit strange cities
That knew "recession" before we were born,
That are still poor,
To visit squats for strange weekend parties
Where no one really knew anyone;
Steal hallucinogenic mushrooms from our friends,
Dance wildly in wild clothes to weird, wild music
And go to bed with at least five men
Whose drug fuelled passion kept us up half the
night,
Though we still maintained the feeling of a small
child

Waiting for a parent, any parent, to tuck us in at
night.
The next morning, we sat and drank tea in their
kitchen
Nonchalantly not talking of the previous night, day,
days, years,
Feeling something that we could not put in to
words
But if we could it would probably have been,
"Weird."

Time was
Time was

Time was we would invite people to our house for
Birthday, graduation, end of term, someone new
moving in, Anyreason, parties
And lock ourselves in our room
With our very very close, very special friends
Feeling special, inventive;
Inventing strange inventive rituals to celebrate our
inventiveness,
Then spend the next morning painting over our
bedroom walls
With last night's drug induced hallucinogenic
cartoons,
Leaving them for the next tenants to wonder at
And paint over, with white or magnolia.

Time was
Time was

# FIRST BOOK

Time was Star Trek, Dr Who and the Avengers
Did not really exist,
TV was a figment of someone else's imagination
Our own lives having enough excitement anyway.

Time was

Time was we slept with our friend's lover's brother,
And then we slept with our friend
When once we found ourselves alone together,
Unusually drunk, intoxicated, morose and strange
It cheered us up, and he wearing his best friend's,
lover's dress:
Him having slept with her the week before.

Time was we would offer foot massages
To the ones we fancied and only them
Not knowing the words that suggested
The space between the tea cup and the bed
We would be there, together
In my bed, his bed or in a friend's
Having stayed at their house long after supper
was over.

Time was
Time was

Time was mornings didn't exist at all and
Afternoons were subdued, slow, resentful affairs,
Picking up speed as the evenings found us
excited,

Briskly walking through the park seeing street
lights
Scintillating through the trees, bought to our
attention
By the rising tide of the hallucinogens ingested
with a six o'clock tea,
Not knowing whose house or chance party
We might later chance upon.

Time was, "On reflection," was a phrase not
known to us
Deep discursive conversations upon the patterns
of our lives
Were habits to be developed twenty years hence
And, "Living in the here and now," meant
Wilfully ignoring last nights unfortunate pleasures
And the weirdness of the last five minutes, for the
excitement of
The next five to come.
The neighbours were strangers from outer space,
Our mothers, weird beyond comprehension
And our own dear fickle friends the centre
Of our small and all important universe.

Time was we lived in Outer Mongolia,
The rest of the world lived in France,
And we all lived on the same street.

Time was, time expanded to encompass the
whole universe,
Contracted to a point between the window pane in
our living room

# FIRST BOOK

And the Sartre filled bookcase, burnt with joss
sticks and cigarettes.

Time was,
Time was,

Time was the pattern of our lives changed from
The evening to the next morning,
Our friends meant everything to us;
And yet we did not know what our friends meant to
us,
Condoms had not been invented, AIDS did not
exist,
God was not in his Heaven,
All had never been well with the world and never
would be.

And yet:

Time was
Time was
Time was,

A la Recherché du Temps Perdu,

Time was.

_____
All play and no work makes John a dole boy.
_____

## PROZAC WARS

I turn the corner of awkward silences
To the room of gossip and discontent.


## DEADLY BOREDOM

Ennui is a state best experienced by teenagers who, on reading the repeated refrain, "And Death shall have no dominion," think they have known death and it is to be found on languid Sunday afternoons after a three course Sunday Lunch. The central course of this lunch consists of roast beef, roast potatoes, roast parsnips, greens, gravy and horseradish sauce. With soup and steamed pudding at either end. Then, after washing up there is nothing: nothing to do, nothing to see, smell, hear, apart from grass growing, tree leaves slowly dying, preparing for the autumn in several months time.

People sit around in stunned silence, reading books, newspapers, recipe cards, with no interest in the content except to wall out all others: human information used to inflict a delicate masochism.

They silently transmit the irritant message, "I am alone and you are not to be bothered with. Not to be indulged, best left alone - ignored." Eventually, like a recalcitrant fly you will go away, fade.

# FIRST BOOK

Go away, fade.

Ennui is a state best experienced by teenagers, who, on reading the repeated refrain, "And Death shall have no dominion," think they have experienced it already.

## CLAUSE 28 - YOU WHAT?

Death to the homophobes
Death to the homophobes
Death to the homophobes

And I shall be loved by a beautiful man

For they live sad and lonely, bigoted lives
For they live sad and lonely, bigoted lives
For they live sad and lonely, bigoted lives

And I shall be loved by a beautiful man

Death to the homophobes
Death to the homophobes
Death to the homophobes

Die, die, die

And I shall be loved by a beautiful man
And I shall be loved by beautiful men
And I shall love beautiful men
And I shall love a beautiful man

And we are the most beautiful of men
And we shall make beautiful love.


## WORD SALAD

"Word Salad," is a symptom some psychiatrists
assign to some       "schizophrenics".
It means a jumble of words that seemingly have
no meaning.
Yet they may be spoken with great emotion:
        tears, rage, fear or occasionally love.
Yet if the jumble of words is attentively listened to,
Questioned, in a firm but friendly manner
Then a certain poetry may emerge.
And often, with further attentive listening
This poetry may subside to reveal
The commonplace stanzas:
Late giros, noisy neighbours, uncaring landlords,
unfaithful lovers,
Library books to be returned, shopping lists.
The so called "schizophrenic" moves on.
While I, the attentive critic,
Wait for the next fascinating individual
To pour fourth their avant-garde tales.

# FIRST BOOK

## CREATING THE FAERIE PALACE: JUST FOR ONE NIGHT

A calm comes to the land of Lauriston, it sleeps and dreams of Party Time.

The little boy elves dress for an evening of high partying in borrowed glitter and delicious PVC: shorts and skirts and pearls and pinnies. We see proud grannies looking on from the cornices: spectral, promising, encouraging. And our impish elves know they are naughty and revel in their ancestor's doting love.

Not so much gin soaked as gin spattered - a light patina of biting aperitif lights up a Queen's battle-dress in the nouveau-grand hallway. She stoops to pick up some discarded gew-gaw, smiles and shows it to a friend as she places it on the table. The table collects Queenly artefacts as the day wears on. Manqué crown jewels displayed in hopeless abandon on the once tawdry Formica table.

The Elves find recordings of music, proudly ancient and sophisticatedly modern, to play on dated machines. We dance for the audience of ever changing Queens and Elves and Dizzies and the almost Straight Looking: actors, never acting the straight role, instead preferring the wavy and the hazy line. The Faeries dance with and for and in-between each other.

In the borrowed Faerie Palace tonight the ritual of The Fabulous Party creates the sacred Faerie energy. To all outward appearances, they eat highly seasoned toasted snacks, dance, chat of this and that, occasionally gulp rich, strong wine while elegantly dressed and momentarily coiffured. For tonight, in the timeless time of Faerie Land, they feel the energy flow between them. The Faeries, Elves, Queens, Dizzies and Straight Acting Ones know that soon the Faerie Land Party Energy will have it's effect on the Land of Euclid and Newton.

The Queens, Elves, Faeries, Dizzies and especially the Straight Acting Ones know that the land from which they have borrowed to find and make Faerie Land needs their energy; but the land of Euclid and Newton is jealous of their precious Faerie gifts and occasionally wishes to destroy them.

Those of the Straight Land, those who claim they are the sole owners of the land, for whom all others live in sufferance, they, in their jealousy and hatred say that they do not need the magic Faerie Energy; that it does not exist and that the Faeries wish to corrupt them, are dangerous, ill in body and mind. The Faeries, meanwhile, know that the more jealousy they find in the Straight Land the longer they must spend in Faerie Land to create the Magic Faerie Energy that is a potent cure for the Straight World's jealousy.

The Faeries have Allies in the Straight World. The Allies sometimes enter Faerie Land, gently flitting through, playing in the Party Ritual where small breaks in the Euclidean and Newtonian space allow. They know the jealousies that the Faeries face. The Faeries live in the straight world as unofficial refugees.

But for tonight a paradise of flirting and teasing and high heels and prayerful partying rules the land of Lauriston. The faerie palace has been created and magic is woven into the very air.


## DIRECT ACTION

I took a hammer to the bathroom scales,
Oh my,
How much lighter I feel already.

## REST

When he died
I didn't hold his hand
I didn't stroke his hair
I didn't stand back while his family scattered his ashes
I didn't sit in my room and play his favourite records
I didn't look at old photos,
Letters,
Stroke a shirt he had lent me that never got returned.
And when holding another man, other men,
Messing up another man's hair, other men's hair
While lying in on long Sunday Mornings,
Early Friday nights,
Before Saturday tea,
I probably, almost never
Thought of him.


## ZEN IN ART OF FUCKBUDDIE

Put all of it in
All of it, all of it
Put all of it in
All of it in
Put all of it in.

Carry on, in ad for night umm.

# FIRST BOOK

## ON DISCOVERING THAT A FRIEND'S LOVER HAS RECENTLY DIED

It's like, I'd like to comb your hair,
Because stroking it would be too intimate.
It's like, I'd like to hold your fingers,
Because holding your hand would be too restricting.
It's like, I would like to grate carrots, fry mustard seed
And mix it all with lemon juice,
Because cooked food would be too wholesome, not simple enough;
And the raw, sharp, pungent freshness
Would compliment how I see you.
It's like, your raw, sad Calmness
Suits you better that your usual frantic nature.
It's like, almost like, grief suits you,
And perhaps there was some relief in his dying?
It's like, I shouldn't speak these words,
And perhaps we shall never be as close as I would like.
It's like, I'd visit your new flat,
But I know you really need to be alone there now.
It's like, I'd really like you to take care,
And I guess you really are.
It's like, whatever card I send will not be right,
Because I'm a stranger to the end,
But I send it anyway.

## AN ARTIST'S PRAYER - MARK 11

An artist's wares
On sale every day
In the mall at Broadstairs:
Fine Paper creations
In yellow and gold,
Major exhibits and an Ivory Toad.
The public adore them
And spend all their money
On Rothkos and Hepworths
And Pipers and Adderleys.
The Children buy pebbles
Painted most finely
Off delightful street urchins
With degrees in decoration.
The artist's prayers are answered
When their pockets are bulging
And the public know that Broadstairs
Is the place to go cruising.

## SQUIRRELLING

I have a gift for words:
I give them ice cream, wardrobes and toasters.

Oh, the poet's pusillanimous pretentiousness
Makes us puke.
When eating a dictionary
One needs to chew well before swallowing.

# FIRST BOOK

## 10:15PM, SUNDAY EVENING:
## SWINDON TRAIN STATION  TOILETS

A handsome man.
A handsome man
With a winsome smile.
A handsome man with a winsome smile.
A handsome man with a winsome smile
And a big cock.
A handsome man with a winsome smile and a big
cock
who may be friendly.
A handsome man with a winsome smile and a big
cock who may be friendly
But probably not your friend.
A handsome man with a winsome smile and a big
cock who may be friendly but probably not your
friend
And certainly not your lover.
A handsome man with a winsome smile and a big
cock who may be friendly but probably not your
friend and certainly not your lover
But who can be admired.
A handsome man with a winsome smile and a big
cock who may be friendly but probably not your
friend and certainly not your lover but who can be
admired
Whose eyes may accidentally meet your eyes.
A handsome man with a winsome smile and a big
cock who may be friendly but probably not your
friend and certainly not your lover but who can be

admired whose eyes may accidentally meet your eyes
For a maximum of a quarter of a second once every 10 minutes.
A handsome man with a winsome smile and a big cock who may be friendly but probably not your friend and certainly not your lover but who can be admired whose eyes may accidentally meet your eyes,
for a maximum of a quarter of a second once every 10 minutes -
Makes the occasional late night train journey so worthwhile.

## FRAGMENTS

Fragments
A rock hammer smashes off a small section
Fragments
Intricately layered pieces of grey-green slate
Fragments
Millions of years of compressed sediments
Fragments
Thin, sharp-edged segments cut a careless hand
Fragments
From a prehistoric sea
Fragments
Layers of a dead past exposed
Fragments
A million pieces on the sea shore
Fragments

# FIRST BOOK

Intricately observed by the beachcombers there
Fragments


## ANITA, DEBORAH, MICHELLE

Just a poem for the Divine
Just a poem for the Divine
Just a poem for the
Lets, Lets.
Just a poem for the
Just a poem for the
Just a poem
Well,
That's David for you.


## TRANSFORMATION VERITE

Once we had Lord Peter Whimsy,
Now we have Allie McBeal.


## STATEMENT OF PURPOSE

Assonance and dissonance and sillysense,
Rhyme and reason and unreality,
Reason and beauty and herbal tea,
Poetry and motion in confusion,
Silly words, silver fox furs and extended verbs,
Pretty words painted, "for whom we serve:"
Poems.

# THE FIRST TIME

Love crawled through my skin and hit my heart
with a hammer.
I could not concentrate at work that day.

# WE TWO BOYS TOGETHER CLINGING

We two boys together clinging,
Hoping that no one sees us snogging.

In suburban bedrooms all over the land,
Young men hide love letters in their true loves
hand.

Two lads sit holding hands on the back of the bus,
"Come on now," said Allan, "that's enough from
you, Gus."

# PERSECUTION COMPLEX

Lord I am a homosexual
Some people say that I am dreadful,
But I am just a guy who's lonely
Looking for his one and only.

(This should really be a song in a Gershwin/Cole
Porter style. I could have gone on but it was
written at the height of the local Clause 28 debate
and it would only have got rather anti-Christian,

which doesn't seem fair and the rhymes would ever recede. So I stopped at this point....)

## GREY-DAY

I am like a puddle,
Muddied by other people's footsteps.
A child sees it's faint reflection and wishes to stop and play.
Its mother drags it into the shopping centre
Encased in her grey Mac against the rain.

The world is roughened concrete,
I am flattened, I am grey.
Muddy splashes discolour our clothing,
And the traffic is colour-faded, drab, today.

I am like a puddle,
Little eddies cut the surface
Of my shallow, discoloured world.
I am like a puddle
Muddied by people walking by.

## HUNGER

I wandered through the desolated city at night
Looking for people to read bedtime stories to.

## BRIGHTON

We talked of men in his life,
Men not in his life
Men who could be in his life if he....
Men who could be in his life if they.....

We went for tea.


## CUSTOMS AND EXCISE

Excise, excision, circumcision;
To cut away, remove, a decision.
Custom, that which is done, repetition.
Repeating patterns form the past
Repetition.

The decision to excise some of the luxury
To pay for the necessary; the day to day.
To cut away the luxury and the intoxicant
Makes the regular affordable, less decadent.

(I got a new job at the VAT office, a branch of
Customs and Excise; it is a very lowly job, mainly
stuffing envelopes. Now I was going to write more
rhymes on the theme of astute, sober, personal
living and compare it to how the state manages
the exchequer: less drinking, more wholesome
food, less late nights and a bit of exercise for me
and taxes on alcohol, gambling and luxury goods
to provide funds for the NHS, roads, schools,

police and libraries. But I haven't thought through my opinions on this yet and I'm not that good at extended rhymes. Suffice to say, I'm happy enough to be stuffing leaflets for the moment and to write the occasional fumbling line of poetry about my current life circumstances.)

## THE FIRST WEEK OF AUGUST

### Monday
Went to work at the VAT Advice Centre and stuffed envelopes.

Met with fellow envelope stuffer at lunch time in the park and discussed rural development in Africa, micro-loans for small farmers, AIDS education, and the wrongs of genetic engineering for rural Africa. He was well informed being from Kenya and having studied rural development at Reading University.

A Colleague told me he will take Thursday morning off to take his sick mother to hospital.

### Tuesday
Thought about taking the UK government to the European Court of Human Rights for continuing to produce Atomic weapons.

Went to a neighbours birthday party and met a four and a half year old boy called Ben and painted his nails whilst first making sure it was the school holidays.

Played dead lions in the park to calm him down, rediscovering the Zen pleasures of looking at the late evening clouds.

Thought of asking raven haired, sensuous lipped, unshaven thirty year old home to make mad passionate love, or failing that cuddling up on the sofa.

Went home and watched "This Life" on TV.

**Wednesday**

Woke up every morning and looked at the mail on the hall table and wondered if it would carry the news of my fathers death.

Nearly started e-mail war by sending one word reply (the word was *Bitch)* not realising that the Customs and Excise Intranet e-mail system does not understand sarcasm and camp irony.

Sent e-mail to Customs and Excise Local Equal Opportunities Officer to complain about gross and irritating incident of homophobia in the VAT Advice Centre.

Watched "Buffy - Vampire Slayer" on TV.

**Thursday**

Met with the Customs and Excise Reading and Writing Group, there were two of us, I read, "I Am My Own Hero" by John Hoggett, Sue read from Captain Correli's Mandolin, I read "After the Silence There is Silence" by AF Harold.

My line manager tells me that my colleague's mother has died.

Phoned up personal ad in local paper at one pound per minute and realised that if the advertiser phoned back I may have to clean my room.

I cycle around planning cabarets that will never be performed.

Go to the poets cafe at the Rising Sun Arts Centre, write this poem in the break and perform it to amused audience.

**Friday**

Pay reflexologist for therapeutic foot massage.

Collect manuscript of new poetry book from proof reader Matthew.

Realise my cooking has become boring and repetitive.

## HOW DO YOU COPE WITH WORK

Do you have sex in the loo?
When there's nothing else to do,
With the lovely bosses daughter
And you know you shouldn't oughtta?

Do you send out slanderous e-mails?
About the men at work and the females,
And say, "it's just a way of talking,"
When the boss he comes stalking?

Do you go for team building teas?
Bounce soft toys upon your knees,
Eat far too much cake and chocolate,
Because you're feeling fraught and desolate?

## STREET WISDOM

You don't have to work here, it's mad. Help!
You don't have to help here but it works -  Mad!
You don't have to work here to help, it's mad.
You don't have to work..................

I knew I shouldn't have had that third rum and black last night.

## WORK IS A CURSE IN VERSE

WAH!
Cooped up in this rat hole
With people so mediocre I shrink,
Then expand again to three times my natural size to compensate.

Paul sits there quiet, sensible,
Smiles occasionally, thinking of private pleasures.
Quite right too,
'Cause anything anyone says around here will be picked;
Picked up, picked on, picked apart, picked.
Pick, Peck, Pick,
Battery chickens disconsolately tearing at each others plumage,
Peck, pick, peck;
Then we sit quiet again and we stare at our screens

# FIRST BOOK

Pick, peck, pick, peck, pick.

And as for the others,
Well we indulge in racy racist jokes.
Then quickly laugh and smile,
Challenging like,
As if to say, "I'm only joking, challenge me if you dare!"
We know the company policy
But the manager's a hypocrite, makes Irish jokes about Declan,
So she can't tell him off then can she?
And her manager tells anti-Italian jokes
While mentioning the company anti-bullying policy.
She, meanwhile, thinks of her Italian mother and gently seethes,
Then makes more anti-Irish jokes about Declan.
Besides, this verbal war of attrition
Compensates for the boredom of the job.

Once they made, "Witticisms," about certain Asian religions.
I, with rocket speed wit retorted,
"It's not them I have the problem with, it's the Christians!"
Just to shake them into some sense of proportion.
Not sensible really,
But if I object I get accused of, "Political correctness."

Trouble is, if they find out that I may publish this

I'd get accused of breaking the clerical conduct policy
And I've had a verbal warning already.
You just can't win,
You just can't win.


## SONG OF THE FAT BOY

Stupid, stupid, stupid, stupid.
"Fat!" she said.
"You're fat."
Stupid, stupid, stupid sneering thin girl.

"Fat boys eat too much,"
"Fat boys are out of control,"
"Fat boys wear ugly clothes,"
"Fat boys - breath in - hold it - don't move,"
"Fat boy, heart attack in waiting,"
"No lover and .................."

"Don't wear that, you'll look fatter."

Listen, thin girl, at least I don't stick my finger down my throat in the loo after supper,
And go to aerobics 'till I ache,
Stare at pancakes with ice cream with self-denying longing.

And what about my health?
I'm a health risk, you say,
In your bullying way,

# FIRST BOOK

Yet you sit in a pub drinking beer, G & T,s and
vermouth
While inhaling other people's smoke.
I didn't ask to come to this pub
And you don't catch me drinking till I sway,
Yet you think you can lecture me this way.

Get a life stupid thin girl.
Stupid, stupid, stupid, stupid.

As far as I can see driving a car is a much bigger
risk than being fat.
Fumes from cars cause people to die from asthma
and bronchitis
And the fumes are worse in a car,
All of us knows someone who has been in a car
crash,
Yet who goes, "Ugh, car driver, only nasty people
drive cars!"
And are casualty departments filled with people
hurt by falling fat people?
I think not.

Fat people do no harm to anyone but themselves,
But perhaps that will change if I hear any more
comments form you.

## INCOMPREHENSIBLE

You know
I don't really understand straight men
But then
I wouldn't really want to.

## CHANGING THE WORLD

If I were to write a book called, "Changing The World,"
It would have a recipe for chocolate cake
With instructions on inviting one hundred strangers around to taste it,
And make strong suggestions for getting their own favourite recipes in return.

It would have instructions on holding convocations of school children
To ask them what would be the most appropriate punishments for parents who slap, snarl and beat,
And give instructions for Non Violent Direct Action
Where children can learn the tactics of naming and shaming,
Making banners, invading offices and using mobile phones to contact their lawyers.

I would instruct soap opera makers
To include story lines where Ken Barlow
Leeds a radical faction of Amnesty International

# FIRST BOOK

In invading the local engineering works that
manufacture torture instruments for use in
America and China's prisons.
Ken would lead the group in smashing them with
domestic hammers.
The Rovers Return would become a theme pub
for homecoming revolutionaries.

I would give instructions on what presents to give
your lawyer
After he has taken the Government to task for
their latest misdemeanours,
Organic champagne, home grown strawberries
and a favourite Chocolate cake recipe never go
amiss.

My book, called, "Changing The World"
Would have poems, party games, origami
instructions, paper aeroplane folding instructions,
And suggestions for successful tree planting.

I would give instructions on holding impromptu
comedy festivals
Outside the houses of those that advocate
flogging, hanging and the bringing back of the
birch
To encourage community participation in the
assessment of gentle mocking humour as a
revolutionary tool.
I would encourage the melding of the work of
Kenny Everet, Jennifer Saunders and the Goons

With the work of Marx, Engels, Goldman, Pankhurst and Tatchell.
"All humour to the Soviets," would be one of my chapter headings.
By writing my book
I might not feel that I was changing the world
But that I had encouraged a few dedicated and wonderful souls.

But instead I will sit in this cafe,
Drink tea,
And watch the world go by.
Oh look, over there goes another handsome young man on a microscooter,
And over there I can just make out some stragglers from the latest riot outside the WTO talks,

How grand the world seems today.


## RELAX, REJUVENATE, RENEW

I will sit back, and like a child watching a picture book unfold on a parents lap at bedtime, I will watch the world unravel before my very eyes.

# FIRST BOOK

---

Statement of derision, delight, embarrassment, celebration, defiance; Accusatory, explanatory defamation; incendiary exclamation; Exhalation; demanding, attention seeking declaration:

## POOF

---

## WALK

Under the trees is the earth.
Beside the wood is the stream.
Above the stream is the grass.
In the grass is the skull.

> Leafy tree.
> Wet stream.
> Green grass.
> Dead skull.

Each has a story,
Each begs a question,
The skull speaks the loudest,
"How did I die?"

Under the trees is the earth,
Beside the wood is a stream,
Above the stream there is grass,
In the grass is a skull.
I am walking with friends.

## STOP THE SOLDIERS

One of my managers at work said that the May Day protesters from last year, the Millennium, had offended people by graffitting on the Cenotaph. They had daubed, "don't glorify war." She said that the soldiers were all some mother's son. But I say that any mother worth her salt would cry and rant and rave the moment any son or daughter of hers joined the armed services and then, having cried and ranted and raved for long enough, mount a picket outside their local recruiting offices to try and stop any more young fools joining these so called services.

Surely everyone knows that the point of the Army, Navy and Airforce is to kill or to be killed?  They get trained in handling and using guns and stuff - stuff that kills - and other people are trained in using stuff to kill them.

It's not as if they get trained in defusing conflicts, calming things down and sorting it all out. I don't suppose they get trained in going, "Ere, what's wrong with you then?"  I expect they get trained in killing people and I expect that they get told that it is unlikely they will get killed because, "We have better defences than they do," and I expect that's what, "The other side," gets told too.

So come on now, don't expect me to be sympathetic when a soldier dies, I'm more likely to say, "Well what did you expect?" Besides, don't all those dead soldiers deserve more than a good cry and then sending off more? Wouldn't a better memorial be to shut down the recruiting offices?

I remember painting, "Don't work for this firm," outside my local Army Recruitment office, isn't that a more fitting memorial than the Cenotaph with it's pompous slogan?

Come on now all you mothers, make a banner, invade a recruiting office, save a few future sons that my manager was so concerned about.


## WINDOWLESS IN EXCELSIS

Defenestration,
Smash, smash, smash, smash, smash,
May Day in Oxford Street.


## THE SIMPLY DIVINE

When Jesus was still God
How certain we were in our diversities;
The bright, gaudy drama of Catholic homophobia
With the quiet grandeur of the homely Baptist Chapel.

## EPISTEMOLOGY

We only know wet
Because there is dry.
We only know life
Because there is death.
We only know beauty
Because there is ugliness.
We only know pretty
Because there is witty and pretty and bright,
Because there is boring and ugly and dull.
We only know, "To have,"
Because there is, "To have not."
Though sometimes we have the stars!

## QUEERSPACE

In Queerspace anything can happen
Physicists talk of bent space
But in Queerspace it is bent already.

## EPIPHANY

I
I don't
I don't want
I don't want to
I don't want to go

# FIRST BOOK

I don't want to go to
I don't want to go to bed
  don't want to go to bed
      want to go to bed
         to go to bed
            go to bed
               to bed
                  bed

## A CONTENTED LIFE

They asked him the secret of a long life,
"Leave the most difficult things 'til last," he said.
Breathing his last.

He was fifty.

Quite a good to age to go;
As he quite possibly thought.

## FATHER FIGURE

There came a time in middle age when I realised I smelt like my father: A strange mixture of stale, damp hay and old kitchen smells.

# A HISTORY OF HETEROSEXUALITY

Get married, flirt with your potential sister in law on the night before your wedding. Bury the wife, get a new one the next week. Obsessively eye up women on the beach, using Zies binoculars in front of the wife and children and call it bird watching. Buy "contact" magazines, put in an ad or two, persuade the wife to join in.
Leave the old man because he's obsessed with sex. Run off with a man who has just left his wife. Get pregnant by the new boyfriend, have an abortion. New boyfriend runs off with best friend. Put personal ad in dating mag. Meet new women, invite them to dinner, insult them by cooking cream laden food and then saying, "Don't eat too much or you'll get fat". Have children, bring them up, treat them badly, then ignore them. Die, have it said at your funeral that you were a role model to your children, wonderful husband, caring and dedicated wife with a talent for mothering, always there when they needed you, a pillar of the community.


## CODE BREAKING

I blasted out, accusingly.
I spoke in mock-manic ranting.
She said with soothing exasperation.
She questioned, brooking no idiocy this time.
I sniffed in mock-childish, sulky, humility.

# FIRST BOOK

A mildly uncomfortable silence reigned for half a minute.

She questioned, half haughtily, testing the water, seeing if normality was rearranged and resumed.
I replied, sinking into the comfortableness of unresolved questions, hopeful that the conversation would take a more realistic turn.

"You bastard,"
"I'm a bastard,"
"Sit yourself down and have a nice cup of tea,"
"What's wrong?"
"Nothing,"

A mildly uncomfortable silence reigned for half a minute.

"Well now, a piece of cake?"
"Hm, that'd be nice,"

"You bastard," I blasted out, accusingly.
"I'm a bastard," I spoke in mock-manic ranting.
"Sit yourself down and have a nice cup of tea," she said with soothing exasperation.
"What's wrong?" she questioned, brooking no idiocy this time.
"Nothing," I sniffed in mock-childish, sulky, humility.

A mildly uncomfortable silence reigned for half a minute.

"Well now, a piece of cake?" she questioned, half haughtily, testing the water, seeing if normality was rearranged and resumed.
"Hm, that'd be nice," I replied, sinking into the comfortableness of unresolved questions, hopeful that the conversation would take a more realistic turn.

## DRAMA – THESIS

Ah, you young men who cut your wrists
Friends running after you
Bandages in hand.
How exciting you make life.

## NIGHT OF THE LIVING DEAD

Become a person for me.
Tell me stories of yourself,
Put a twinkle in your eye,
Smile at me,
Ruffle my hair,
Let me ruffle your hair.
Smile me a bitter little smile.
Scowl.
Come into my house, ignore me.
Look away and grit your teeth when I look at you.

# FIRST BOOK

Go to your room when I leave mine.
Leave, leaving no forwarding address.
And at night I dream of you
Holding me close.
Hold me close,
Hold me closer,
Hold me close.
And we are the living dead.


## HOUSEHOLD CHORE

Trapped in the twilight world of Tesco's,
Light levels never changing,
Wandering eternally,
Never finding the thing I want.
The only delight, the sight of children
Inappropriately exploring cardboard boxes
Or driving their parents to distraction
By dropping small items of food.
How I long to pick them up, hand them back to the
child,
See them drop them, pick them up again,
Repeat the action twenty times more
Until we are both tired of it.
But no, instead I scour the almost completely
unfamiliar shelves
Looking for Tesco own brand baked beans.
The vast prison walls crowd in.

## STREET WISDOM – FOR DAMIAN AND GARY

It's never too late to have a misspent youth.

## PSYCHOBABBLE

"I wonder if that's projection?"
He said,
As I smacked him round the gob,
"Probably," I said,
As he skidded across the floor.
But it still felt good.

## A BLESSING – TO BE USED AT CHRISTENINGS, BIRTHDAYS, COMING-OUT AND RETIREMENT PARTIES

Do lots of things I would never dream of doing.

## THE STORY IS A FORM  BASIC TO HUMAN BEINGS

The beginning
The middle
The end

The beginning

The beginning

# FIRST BOOK

The middle
The end

The middle

The middle, the middle, the middle, the middle

The beginning
The middle
The end

The end.


## THE MORAL HIGH GROUND

Between the High Moral Principle
And the Lowest Common Dominator
Lies the Middle Ground.


## DIVINITY 3

I am god
Which explains
Nothing
Really.

## CONFRONTATIONS

I want to meet the man of my nightmares,
Stare him in the face, and say,
"What the hell do you think you're doing."


## GRIEF AND MOURNING

It's difficult to change your life
Except when you grow old and die,
And that's just going with the flow.
So go on, do it anyway.


## COLLATERAL DAMAGE

I am the collateral damage of my parents divorce.
"Don't mind me," I should have said
As they sniped and bickered across of our kitchen,
One time attempting murder,
Another, indulging in multiple affairs.

Alcohol fuelled depression
Made my environment toxic.

Time to go, I think
And wander round the woods,
Have the gentle breezes
Wash away their psychic soot.
Be inspired by the spring shoots
Gently unfolding from long winter dormancy.

# FIRST BOOK

Flowers coming soon I expect.
And above, the odd migratory bird flies on by.


## CONFIDENTIALLY YOURS

The trouble with knowing poets
Is the constant risk of ending up in one of their
poems.
I even ended up in one of my own poems once.
There I was, just this character drifting across a
page.
Oh!
And I was planning quiet, personal anonymity.
Safe,
For the rest of my life,
Safe.
Now just what was the author thinking of?
I'd sue him
But I don't think I can afford it.
That's the trouble with poets,
So honest,
In a sneaky, yet so in your face sort of way.
Oh well.


## THE BANALITY OF EVIL

The bri-nylon cushion covers,
"Eastenders" on the TV.
The beat up old Volvo
In the tarmac yard

Of a suburban maisonette.
Mothers with push chairs and toddlers.
And elderly people,
Staggering a little,
Passing on through.
This is the banality of evil.


## I AM STARING INTO SPACE WITH MY EYES CLOSED

I am staring into space with my eyes closed.

I am staring into space with my eyes closed and I see so much.

I am staring into space with my eyes closed and I see so much
Space is infinite in here.

I am staring into space with my eyes closed and I see so much
Space is infinite in here

With my eyes open my world is so small.

I am staring into space with my eyes closed.

I am staring into space with my eyes closed.

## UNTITLED 9

I hate the world and the world hates me,
Twiddly twiddly twiddly twiddly dee.


## THE COMPENSATIONS OF PHILOSOPHY

There is nothing in the world that is perfect
There is nothing in the world that is
There is nothing in the world that
There is nothing in the world
There is nothing in the
There is nothing in
There is nothing
There is
There
There there
There there there
There there there little child
There there
There
There there
There there there
There there there little child
What do you want for your tea?

## PROFESSIONAL CODES OF ETHICS AND PRACTISE

It takes three years to be a hairdresser
And seven for a doctor
But there's no training for poets.
My God!
Think of the harm you could do.


## THE WILD AND SCUZZY DAYS OF YOUTH

Dancing on fridges in kitchens at parties on the Junction in the eighties;
Waking with hash hangovers on the floor in living rooms under tenth hand, unwashed sleeping bags, seeing the boyfriend of the woman who is a housemate as he wakes and he rolls in my arms as I turn towards him then she walks in as we hug for the moment is the thing and the silence is uncomfortable and comfortable as my life is.


## LIFESTYLE RESEARCH QUESTIONNAIRE

"Sex or drugs or rock and roll?" she professionally inquired.
"Rock and Roll," I confidently replied.
"It's good healthy exercise, always coming back into fashion,"
"You can meet a variety of people for social intercourse"

# FIRST BOOK

"And who knows, it might even lead to the other two!"

## THE DEGREES OF INTIMACY

How wonderful it is – boom boom.
How wonderful it is – boom boom.
How wonderful it is,
When someone new comes into your home,
Examines all your records,
All your books,
And transforms all your tat
Into objets trouves
By their fascinated gaze.
Then they undo all your buttons,
One by one,
Taking off all your clothes,
Stand back,
Look,
And smile.

## MODERN ART

"This Art is Modern,
It makes no sense.
It's big and bold and brassy,
Big blobs of paint on a big, big canvas
In a big gallery
And it costs a lot of money.
It doesn't make any sense,

Just like this poem.
My eight year old could have painted the picture,
And I could have written this poem.
It's got no rhyme, no rhythm,
And God knows what he's on about?
It's not even pretty,
It doesn't look good on the page.
What's the point of it?
Just like that picture,
What's the point of that then?
Just big dollops of paint on an effin' huge canvas.
What's the point of that then?
Just like this poem.
Just like this poem.
I don't understand modern poetry me,
It's all a meaningless jumble of words,
That's what.
I mean, at school we had Siegfried Sassoon
And all those war poets
But what are this lot on about?
And at school the girls had skipping rhymes,
And us boys counted, "Spuds."
"One potato, two potato,"
That way you knew who was "it".
And they had rhyme, all those skipping games.
"One potato, two potato," lots of rhythm.
Lots of rhythm there.
But all this modern stuff
It's got none of that.
It's just words on a page,
And not many of 'em either,
Just simple words thrown on a page.

# FIRST BOOK

What they on about?
Makes no sense.
It makes no sense.
It makes no sense to me mate.
Absolutely no bleedin' sense at all.
Why can't they write proper poems
About blood and guts and war and death,
And losing your mother,
And falling in love,
And the corn blowing in the wind
On the Oxfordshire plain.
You know, like when you see it
Driving down from the Chilterns,
Driving towards Didcot or somewhere?
Why can't they write about that then?
With rhymes!
And rhythm!
Why can't they do that then eh?
I mean, Art is Art,
And words are words,
And big blobs of paint are just big blobs of paint.
And blobby words just smeared over a big bit of paper
Are just blobby words
Looking lost on a big bit of paper.
What am I supposed to make of that then?
I don't know.
You comin' down the pub?"

## POETRY WORKSHOP

I took my poem,
Slagging modern poetry off,
To the poet's café.
They slagged it off
Mercilessly.
The irony was not lost on me
Or my adoring audience.

## THIS IS MODERN ART

Buttons,
Wordblobs,
Radiating
Mudclouds.

## WAR IN THE PEACE GROUP

I think I've said enough already.

## EMPTINESS

The slinging of unfortunate and outrageous arrows
Stopped:
They came to an end
As we all realised that what we wanted
We would never,

# FIRST BOOK

Somehow,
Win.


## THE POWER CENTRES OF THE WORLD ARE TO BE FOUND IN THE PUBLIC TOILETS

I sit and listen
To the sound
Of piss hitting stainless steel
And think,
In my ignorance of women,
That this
Is a manly sound.


## CHRISTMAS

Presence
And presents,
Wrapping and unwrapping,
The joy of choosing for someone,
Weighing them up so carefully.

Find childhood memories of wonder:
Santa may or may not come down the chimney?
But wrapped presents are there in the morning.

And Daddy tried to strangle mummy.
Oh,

Years of dust,

And dust,
Years of arid dust,
Tasting in the mouth.

Empty people, and bitter too.
Stone;
Cut and splut and saw and dust,
Cut by angle grinders producing dust clouds.

The family.


**SIMON**

Ah, a boy.
A boy whose eyes smile,
A boy whose eyes smile in my direction.
And where else is there to look,
Except into his?


**THE GOLDEN AGE OF POP**

The time is now.
Always the time is now.
The always time is now.
The time always is now.
The time is always now.
The time is now always.
Now is the time.

# FIRST BOOK

## THE WAR POETS

I read a book called, "Deafness,"
And it said, "Where are the war poets?"
Well, last night I had a nightmare.
Woke up screaming,
(Or was I just snoring loudly?)
Worried that I would wake someone up.
In the room below me
Someone dreamed the USA had made a mistake,
That one of their bombers had gone astray
And bombed Bristol by mistake.
Why Bristol?
Perhaps because that's where his friend, Paul, lives?
He woke up screaming, "What the fuck's going on?"
But that was because the Sikh's were celebrating Vaisakhi.
The temple's just across the road
And they were singing loudly, through microphones,
Celebrating the spring.
Some Muslim's gather in the park
Carrying placards that say,
"Don't end the war except through Islamic politics.
I cycle to Cyberspice, my local Asian internet café.
My friend William is in Saudi Arabia, picking up handsome men.
Am I a tourist in my own town?
And how do wars end?

## FRAGMENT – 1

French knitting
      Skipping
      Kissing
      It's a progression.

## FRAGMENT – 2

Art
Flame
Fame
Tart

## FRAGMENT – 3

What do you do when your friend
Gets off with the guy you fancy?
Do you stamp your feet
And throw a great big Nancy?
Do you............
      (Oh, I can't be bothered to go on…)

# FIRST BOOK

## FRAGMENT – 4

The first night I met him
He was in silk.
All in silk,
All in silk,
Bloody Hell,
He blew my horn like Acker Bilk.
Down in the valley,
Where the green grass grows.

## FRAGMENT – 5

It must be spring;
Mr pale face, hunky youth
Is on his balcony again.

## KEROUAC

He was the original Hipster,
Throwing words at the dart target
Of American Neo-liberalism:
In pre-Vietnam innocence,
When Korea raged, and naked spirituality
Collided with heavy drugs.

## AMERICAN ENGLISH POETRY

I hate the waiters that make you feel special
And then go on and do it to everyone else too.
I hate the waiters that smile as they eat you,
Who ask how you are,
Say how wonderful it is to see you,
And then say it to everyone else too.
Coffee, croissants, guacamole and a smile,
That's a very large, and very winning smile.
Oh sweetheart, butter my teacake,
Then move on and put margarine on someone else's.
I'll sit in the window – eat and read the Guardian.
See you next week honey,
And mine's a latte-grand, skimmed milk and not too strong,
No cake, I'm not really watching my figure
But my cholesterol's a little high.
See you next week,
Tell me I'm special,
Smile very winningly.
You do it so well Mickey,
You do it so goddamned well.

# FIRST BOOK

## TEASING MEMORIES

Yeah, double-glazing salesmen:
No one really likes them, do they?
Except this woman I knew,
She asked one in, with her housemates.
You know, just being friendly,
And they had a bottle of wine or two,
Invited him in for dinner,
Laughed, joked, had a fabulous time.
One of the best evenings ever,
Just her, her house mates, and a double-glazing salesman.
But then, it was the eighties,
And she was a community worker,
And that's what they do.
Throw parties, invite loads of people, get them to talk to one another.
Have a really great time:
Community workers, in the eighties.
And have friends who, with cuts all up their arms.
Self inflicted, self harm,
Self harming.
Always joking, always smiling,
With scars on her arms.
And her friend, the community worker,
Befriending her, propping her up,
Staunching the despair,
The despair that never showed,
Just the scars on her arms.
That's what it was like,
Knowing community workers,

In the eighties.
She was always there,
Close,
Friendly,
Always there,
Encouraging, friendly, a right laugh.
Said, she was giving her friend a couple of years,
Like she was giving up herself for a couple of years.
For her friend.
Staunching the wounds.
Healing the scars.
Though they're always there of course.
A couple of years.
With the cuts, the scars, the self, self harm.
But that's what it was like,
Knowing community workers,
Who were such good fun,
In the eighties.


## I CELEBRATE MY INDEPENDENCE

One day, when I was a young man, aged twenty-five or so,
I met some friends and I said,
"I want to be married."
Not that there was anyone, male or female,
Who I wanted to settle down with.
Just that desire for a big party.
Wedding presents, cards, a dressed up Rolls Royce,

# FIRST BOOK

And all for me.
Paid for by my family.

You see, it never really happened for me,
No big twenty-first birthday party,
No huge, all day and half the night
Father paid, I designed,
Party.
It never happened,
Never happened.

So I'm gonna celebrate my independence.,
Have a big party,
Invite relatives and friends from around the region,
From Bridlington, Solihull and Didcot
To a big room.
With cream table cloths with discreet patterns
And Champagne and a big cake,
To celebrate my independence.
Where Aunties and cousins have spent all
afternoon
Making an immense finger buffet,
The men seeing to the wine list and the parking.

And there's a disco with lots of 70's hits,
And Annie Lennox, Boyzone, S-Club, Tatu and
The Cheeky Girls,
Where young boys, aged seven or eight,
Sons of cousins, and sons from uncles' second
marriages,
Wear oversized, velvet bow-ties,

And eat cocktail cherries, given to them by indulgent aunties.
And we'd celebrate,
Celebrate my independence.

You see my lovers never lasted very long,
They were strange, weekend and holiday affairs.
With passion, yes, but never for very long,
A year or two at most,
And even then, only at the weekends.
So I'm celebrating my independence.

And there'll be presents,
For everyone to see and gawp at.
And all wrapped in a rain forest's worth of shiny paper,
An Argos catalogue's worth of presents,
Half a Habitat catalogue,
And a smattering of high tech Ikea oddities,
A selection of Fairtrade handicrafts
And an antique toasting fork,
Yes, and all to celebrate my independence.
And the children will eat until they're nearly sick.

Elderly uncles and aunts will dance for the first time in years,
Friends will congratulate me for having such a smashing idea.
And you see, we were celebrating my independence.

And towards the end of the evening

# FIRST BOOK

A young, not so young, almost middle aged,
decidedly middle aged    man,
Eyes me up,
Chats to me,
Leans in.
We dance, hold hands,
Snog.

We're celebrating my independence,

We go home, to my place
Snog some more.

We have breakfast and he goes home,
Because, you see,
I'm celebrating my independence.

## BIRTHS, MARRIAGES, DEATHS

Men holding  babies at funerals.
Men holding  babies at funerals;
Flowers,
A beautiful chapel,
A woman made ugly by grief,
And a boy,
A young lad, tasting grief, and it was too strong.
And men holding babies at funerals.
Babies always cry at weddings,
But they're quiet at funerals.
Middle aged men hold their babies at their friend's
funeral.
Men holding babies at funerals.

*John Hoggett*

# A BEARD IS A CUSHION TO BE LEANED ON

Well I met a man in the street in Oxford and he asked me if I knew of any good pubs and I said I had come from one just now and he said, no, not just any old pub but a really good one with lots of women and I exclaimed: I don't know, I'm a dedicated homosexual! And he said, looking a bit puzzled: Oh, I don't know about that, and I said, what are you doing in Oxford? And he said he couldn't tell me and so I asked again, and he said he was on a parachute course so I thought he was probably a squaddie, age about 27. And then he said, have you ever been to Thailand? And I said no and he said ……… And before he could say much his friend came along, in the street see, him and his friends, out on the town, in a busy street, in Oxford at 9 o'clock on a Friday night, when visiting to do a parachute course, looking for a loud pub with lots of women. And his friend said, come on, we've got to go, crossing his arms, legs well planted taking no nonsense, sort of stance and said, is he trying to chat you up? Like they had been through this before or something? And I shook his hand, the dark haired one who looked as though he was in charge of the three of them, I said, handing his friend back to him, get drunk, have a good time and look after each other, and then I turned to the one who had spoken to me, the one who had been to Thailand, the one who did not know about that, the one who had looked intrigued and confused and pleased by something, someone, some people in Thailand, and I put my hand out and shook his hand and put my arms around him and he LEANED IN, and HIS HEAD LEANED ON MINE, LEANED ON MY SHOULDER, LEANED ON MY BEARD, CUSHIONED ON MY BEARD and HE LEANED IN and I STROKED HIS HAIR and then I stopped, not wanting to get him in trouble with his friends, in a street in Oxford at 9 o'clock  at night, not knowing what they thought, not wanting to stop, wanting to hold him some more, STROKE HIS HAIR, FEEL HIM LEAN INTO ME, INTO MY BEARD, HIS HEAD CUSHIONED ON MY BEARD. I stopped and looked at him and he said: Thank you, thank you, thank you for that, and he looked at me, straight at me and I looked at him and said goodbye and I walked away and I felt torn up inside.

## THE STRANGENESS OF IT ALL

The strangeness of
Looking at people on the train and looking
Away before they look at you and then
Realising that they are probably doing it to you
too.

*John Hoggett*

# WHAT MAKES YOU FIT TO BE A POET?

Maybe it's having a daddy who recited nursery rhymes at bedtime, while bouncing you on his knee?

Maybe it was the boys at school, young footbally lads, who dissyingly switched the letters in common-day phrases, so that, "Wet paint," became, "Pet waint," and, "John Hoggett," became, "Hon Joggett?"

Or maybe it was hearing that well educated academic lady saying that iambic pentameters have the rhythm of the heart and the length of the breath; and later, finding out that old windbag Ginsberg had a particularly long breath and that a meter is the length of a particularly long step but that metre is the rhythm of a poem?

Maybe it was those exciting, long riddle sessions with a young and excitable stepmother that seemed to irritate everyone else (why did the viper vipe her nose? Because the adder 'ad 'er 'ankie!).

Maybe, on thinking back to those fellows at school, who asked, "If you had a band, what would you call it?" Not that any of you were in a band or could even play an instrument - you, twenty-five years later, looking back, would call yours, "The Protonarative Envelope." Thus showing just a smattering of Chomsky while maintaining the pretentiousness of youth.

Was it having enough of a social conscience to want things changed, not enough confidence to

say it out loud, but enough gumption to write
things down?
Or was it reading that the poet Ginsberg, that
druggie, beatnik, pacifist, Buddhist, who was so
prolific, used to write his diary, insert line breaks,
and then send it off to his publisher?
And finally, the gift of most poets, the blessed
discovery that a past it's sell by date love affair
makes for an excellent lyric?


## IMMATURE SEXUALITY

It must be a middle aged thing,
But I've started fancying
Plumbers, electricians, telephone engineers:
Sad I know,
But also, quite exciting.


## BLISS

I want to take lots of drugs and smile a lot.


## BEAUTIFUL

Oh beautiful queer world;
Trees and oceans and men snogging,
Do we love you?
Do we hate you?
Do we destroy  you?

Do we?
Oceans, fish, rivers, trees, rain,
Concrete Jungles, railway yards, transatlantic runways.
And a beach; low, slow waves, rolling in.
Two men rolling in the sand, after dusk, snogging,
Naked, engulfed, oceanic, celebratory.
Engorged and engaged:
Oh beautiful queer world,
Roll on.


## CLIMATE CHANGE POEM NO 1

We are all playing the victim now.


## DO YOU WANT TO SLEEP WITH ME?

Allen Ginsberg used to perform his poems
And if, from stage
He spotted some handsome young man
Who took his fancy
He would shout out,
"Do you want to sleep with me?"
And often enough
These handsome young men would go off to
        Allen's home, or to a hotel, or to the young
        man's home.
The young men, often claimed a gentle and understated heterosexuality.
They would emerge,

# FIRST BOOK

In the morning,
Smiling,
Unharmed,
Charmed
And charming;
Such was the capacity of this original beatnik to
spread love around this fractured world.
His love life may have been chaotic,
His best friend, a tortured, genius, heroin addict
Who accidentally shot his wife in a drunken party
game,
And who constantly belittled his friends;
His lover, a neurotic/psychotic, neo-hetero.
But he always sent the young men home happy,
Spiritually and physically blest,
Touched by fame,
Mainlining Beatnik history.
Sleeping with a man who slept with Kerouac.
Blessed by the spiritual slapper from Patterson.
And me?
I cruise the Guardian Personal adds,
Bored by, "I like gardening, music, walking,"
"I want honesty, friendship, possibly more."

So:    dive into the pool
       dive into the pool
       dive into the pool

Take me on tour,
Give me the microphone,
And I'll take the young men back to the hotel.
But for now,

*John Hoggett*

These are Tilehurst days,
As I perform cut-ups on Guardian Personal adds
And gather my material:
Wanted, steady, reliable,
Must like the cinema,
No heroin addicts or Jazz friends allowed.


## EQUALITY AND DIVERSITY

Label me, label me;
Let me not reach up to your expectation.
Your trust in me is strictly limited,
Appropriately so, you think.
So labelled, not as I am, by many:
Mistaken for the vaguely mediocre,
My skill gaps often not recognized.
Which is just as well, considering,
Job interviews and all that.
I am boxed into a box that is not mine.
Escaping out the back, I seep out,
Lonely at first,
But losing myself into the woods;
Wandering by ponds, heron's nest, lime avenue,
Tilia Europa leaves made sticky lace by aphids bite.
I lose myself in my rural prison,
A relief from the box of labels.

Stupid, useless, bright, clever, talented,
Poet, dramatist, eccentric,
Straight, homosexual, wasted, middle aged,

164

# FIRST BOOK

Queer, able bodied, living with a disability,
Living with it, living with it all,
Special needs, mental health difficulties, low self
esteem:
Embrace the label, repel the labeller;
"Bitchy little man of discernible means,"
"Unnecessary,"
"Getting along. Living with it."

"And how are you?"


## CRUSHINGLY HANDSOME

I always trip over the arrogant art students,
Then try to prove I'm as good as them:
The handsome arrogant ones,
Who decry the bourgeoisie in posh suburban
accents,
Not realizing that fine art is not a working class
thing,
Not the stuff they do anyway.
I name drop some of the artists I know; family and
friends,
He smiles and talks of his Grandfather's abuse of
children.
I mention the art students I knew twenty years
ago,
He said, "It's a sink or swim world,"
"Only the excellent survive."
He said, "Suicide is a selfish thing."
I remember the dead art student.

He decries folk clubs, the Velvet Underground, comedians, sing-a-longs,
But he loves Warhol, because Warhol knew everything and used everyone.
It's like being at school again
And I'm trying to prove I'm as good as them:
But I'm not the head boy,
I don't play rugby,
I won't get four A's in my A' levels,
And I'm just revisiting my past:
Arrogant art students and school boy snobs
Treading on my tender feelings.
So why engage in this battle?
Far better to walk around them,
The arrogant art students,
Because some men are handsome and some of them are charming,
And I like art, it amuses me;
And comforts,
And shocks,
And makes me laugh.


## BOYZ

The happy, smiley young man travels from town to town
To see his friends wow the crowds,
Playing guitars in cafes and bars across the South East.
Flashing white teeth in adoration of songs that tell the stories he knows.

# FIRST BOOK

Driving music that strangers play you on CDs,
In fast cars, as you hitch hike across the rolling hills,
Between Salisbury, Newbury and Woking.
Oh you English youth,
Dancing away in the cafes and bars of England;
Smile in delight at your friends.

## EVENING TIDE

Sitting in bars listening to young men playing guitars
While making subtle bitchy remarks to strangers.
Yes indeed, the simple pleasures really are the best.

## THIS IS THE MODERN WORLD

Two daddies pushing prams through the park together.

## THOUGHTS ON CLIMATE CHANGE, THE G8 CONFERENCE AND ETHICAL FOREIGN POLICIES: JUNE 2005

Isn't it about time we declared war on America?

*John Hoggett*

## LEARNING TO BE A TEACHING ASSISTANT

Metaphors arcing away
Across the assessments and measurements
Of the adult literacy core curriculum.

I sit and freeze with these students
Who get the labels that spell, "Needy,"
"Learning difficulties," "Mental health problems,"
        "English not first language," "shy."
And I sit and hide, wanting to not show
How little I understand what I'm here for.

Metaphors arcing away,
The struggles under a mask of competency,
Students turn up late, leave early, blankly stare,
Flinch, when I offer help;
My skin creeps, and my neck freezes
As I disguise my hiding head.

What is hard for the teacher is hard for the
student.
The black hole of shame for the teaching assistant
Is incomprehensible confusion for the student.

Child sexual assault (vaguely survived),
History of homelessness, fears of racism,
Sometimes understanding bus conductors,
The shame of parent teacher evenings.

The numbness of class echoing the numbness of
psychotropic medication:

# FIRST BOOK

Curriculum reference SLc/E2.1, curriculum reference Wr/E2.1,
Objectives and factual accounts of a learner's abilities
That barely catch the intersecting stories of our lives.

Metaphors arcing away.
Intersecting rainbows of desire,
Likes fishing, cycles everywhere
Persistent troubles with capitals and full stops,
Failed degree (dropped out of university),
Struggling to understand and use conjunctions,
Young children, grown children,
Distinguished amateur artist, just wants to
Hold together a conversation at a party or wedding reception
For Gods sake:
Curriculum reference Ws/E2.2 curriculum reference Ws/E2.1

Metaphors arcing away;
Intersecting rainbows of desire.
What is hard for the teacher is hard for the student:
After six weeks, finally, someone smiles at me.
I am learning to be a teaching assistant for adults learning basic skills.

# 8<sup>th</sup> JULY 2005

Last week I wrote to my mother for the first time in
15 years.
She wrote back,
I didn't open the letter,
You never know what she might say.
Yesterday there were bombs in London.
Tonight I went to the peace vigil.
Racists came and ranted at us:
They calmed down after we listened and
answered their points
With some well thought out arguments.
Even their racism faded,
One talking to our Muslim colleague;
Another left me feeling uncomfortable.
But it was good though,
Bringing a little peace to our corner of the world.
I'm still not opening the letter from my mother.


## JAM

Strawberry poly-bags full, Pick Your Own, squidgy
and cheap, make on hot Sunday afternoons,
sweating in overheated kitchens.

Affectionate
Compassionate
Friendly
Loving
Open                                        hearted

# FIRST BOOK

Sympathetic
Tender
Warm


Serve with home scones and clotted cream, when Granny comes round for tea.

Confident
Empowered
Open
Proud
Safe
Secure

Apricot: Cheap, heated up with water, sieved and used to paste strips of marzipan on to the side of Christmas cake, the remains left congealing in a saucer, ready for children to lick with their fingers before tea time washing up.

Engaged
Absorbed
Alert
Curious
Engrossed
Enchanted
Entranced
Fascinated
Interested
Intrigued

Involved
Spellbound

Marmalade – Silver Shred and Golden Shred on white toast for breakfast.

confused
ambivalent
baffled
bewildered
dazed
hesitant
lost
mystified
perplexed
puzzled
torn

Marmalade – Lime: a strange holiday speciality that maiden aunts and a beloved Gran take from Victorian sideboards.

Vulnerable
Fragile
Guarded
Helpless
Insecure
Leery
Reserved
Sensitive
Shaky

# FIRST BOOK

Marmalade – Tangerine:   simple, exotic luxury to fill up a Saintsbury's shopping trolley.

Disconnected
Alienated
Aloof
Apathetic
Bored
Cold
Detached
Distant
Distracted
Indifferent
Numb
Removed
Uninterested
Withdrawn

Marmalade – Homemade, Seville orange, dark sugar, extra toffee taste, stored in dark cupboards for a month before eating.

Exhilarated
Blissful
Ecstatic
Enthralled
Exuberant
Radiant
Rapturous
Thrilled

Marmalade from the WI market: every Thursday, in the Abbey Baptist Church Hall, all individually labelled by date, type and cook.

Refreshed
Enlivened
Rejuvenated
Renewed
Rested
Restored
Revived

Blackberry: Picked from hedges, squashed into bulging Tesco bags, and later stewed, strained through muslin and finally cooked into a dark red jelly.

Angry
Enraged
Furious
Incensed
Indignant
Irate
Livid
Outraged
Resentful

Gooseberry: Granny H's favourite.

Tense
Anxious
Cranky

# FIRST BOOK

Distressed
Distraught
Edgy
Fidgety
Frazzled
Irritable
Jittery
Nervous
Overwhelmed
Restless
Stressed                                          out

Sugarless:  take equal parts by weight of cooking
apples and cooking dates, put through a Spong
mincer, available at most car boot sales, and mix
with a little lemon juice.  Keep in a fridge for up to
a week.  Can also be served in individual glasses,
topped with yoghurt, vegan yoghurt, for those that
must.


Peaceful
Calm
Clear                                          headed
Comfortable
Content
Equanimous
Fulfilled
Mellow
Quiet
Relaxed
Relieved

Satisfied
Serene
Still
Tranquil
Trusting

Red:    cheap from Tescos, undefined fruit, for winter sandwiches and jam tarts, when it's rent week, the council tax is due and the dole is running thin.

Afraid
Apprehensive
Dread
Foreboding
Frightened
Mistrustful
Panicked
Petrified
Scared
Suspicious
Terrified
Wary
Worried

Mixed Fruit: also from Tescos for everyday dole days.

Annoyed
Aggravated
Dismayed
Disgruntled

# FIRST BOOK

Displeased
Exasperated
Frustrated
Impatient
Irritated
Irked

Crab Apple: a rosy tangerine pink, recipe found in utilitarian library books complete with full plate, colour photographs.

Sad
Depressed
Dejected
Despair
Despondent
Disappointed
Discouraged
Disheartened
Forlorn
Gloomy
Heavy                                    hearted
Hopeless
Melancholy
Unhappy
Wretched

Elderberry and Crab apple:   the best hedgerow folk food, an English secret joy, like local ham and homemade mustard.   Served on home made, whole meal bread, toasted on an old Arga.

Excited
Amazed
Ardent
Aroused
Astonished
Dazzled
Eager
Energetic
Enthusiastic
Giddy
Invigorated
Lively
Passionate
Surprised
Vibrant

Kiwi Fruit: scavenged, from the summer prunings of our gardening colleagues.

Inspired
Amazed
Awed
Wonder

Rose Petal: unbelievable simple, palest pink, aromatic and rare. Collect the petals of twenty scented roses. Melt over a gentle heat, add sugar, and all for one glass jar of sweet scented heaven. Put in fluted glass, seal, wrap with green and silver ribbon, give to ones true love on Lamas Eve.

# FIRST BOOK

Yearning
Envious
Jealous
Longing
Nostalgic
Pining
Wistful

Damson:    served    in    superior    hotels    as    an
accompaniment to muffins as part of the extensive
breakfast.

Disquiet
Alarmed
Disconcerted
Disturbed
Restless
Shocked
Troubled
Uncomfortable
Uneasy
Unsettled


## NEW CRUISING PIECE

The fleet and vigorous young man
Ran up the hill,
Up the hill,
Up the hill,
Into the woods
And sucked me off.

## SCHOOL-WORK-CONTRADICTIONS

"Oh Fuck" said the poet,
"Language!" said the child.

## SLAM

Where does Andrew Motion live?
He says, "Poetry's dead."
He says, "No one reads poetry aloud anymore."
But we, the Poetry Anarchists, aim for the
Annihilation of Boredom.
So lets go round to Andrew M's house,
Megaphone in hand, and reinvent our art form,
The International Radical Slam.

## REDISCOVERING THE MEANING OF LIFE

The patterns of light above a night time curtain,
And what happens when you squint up your eyes,
And these are the important things.

The right way to exhale a cigarette,
And what brand has the coolest aftertaste,
And these are the important things.

The angle of a young man's cheekbones,
And the shadow cast underneath,
And these are the important things.

# FIRST BOOK

## THE THAW

I'm fed up with it,
Fed up with it all.
All the long held grudges and fears,
All the fears.
All those images in my head.
I'm fed up with them all.
Fear of the dead
Who scared me,
Held me frightened.
Fear of the family,
Hateful ghosts,
Frightened of everyone,
I'm fed up with it all.
And all the grudges and all the fears,
All the fears.
But it's all melting,
Like pack ice,
Going south for winter,
Warming up,
Don't know where we're going,
Melting.
The thaw.

*John Hoggett*

## WHAT DOES GAY LIBERATION REALLY MEAN?

Snuggly lesbians:
In da house,
In da house,
In da house.


## PERSONAL COMPUTER

The poem's in the PC,
But is the PC in the poem?
At what future date
Will some academic write a thesis
On, "The first use of the personal computer
As a metaphor in late Elizabethan poetry?"

When Thomas Hardy, in 1915, wrote that
Christmas poem,
About the Ox, the Ass and the Lamb,
Oxen had just about ceased to be used
On the land, on British Farms,
But horses were still used to pull gun carriages.

And personal computers?
The poem's in the PC:
But what use will the PC be in the poetry?

---

Someone turned the scanning electron
microscope upside down. Now I've got RSI.

# FIRST BOOK

---

## EASYJET

My name is Easyjet,
I fly you round the world for the cost of a dole
cheque.
I was born in the brain of a money making
capitalist,
My parents are poverty and luxury.
I live off the oil that burns in my jets.
As I make the world warmer.

I like to entice people to exotic locations,
While sneakily making the world hotter and
dangerous.
I take your children on exciting holidays,
And poison the weather they depend on.
I am young, just a few years old,
I play on old desires of fun, value for money and
excitement.

I am scared of people seeing through my cheap
and tawdry dreams,
Of them seeing my dangerous fumes.
I dream of avarice, of profit, commerce;
A new King in a new counting house, counting out
his money.
I worry about people waking up from their dream,
Of them killing me and not themselves.

*John Hoggett*

## MODERN MANNERS

I hate those people who answer their mobiles while on the loo.

## BAD HABITS

I have this awful habit,
I sing people's phone tunes back to them,
Five minutes after the call.

## UNTITLED 10

How I love the wimpy heterosexual men,
Such companionship and gentle frustration.

## POETIC THOUGHT

I think in Iambic Pentameters.

## PSYCHOSIS - IN TWENTY FOUR HOURS

Strain,
Pain,
Drain;
The pains of the day create an abiding longing.

# FIRST BOOK

Dada,
Surrealism,
Abstract;
Her mind avoids reality, and recreates heaven and hell.

Psychiatrist,
Mother missed,
Blissed;
Hallucinations struggle through the heavy levels of sedation.

Exclaiming,
Explaining,
Sustaining;
It's the little things that push you over the edge.

Crying,
Trying,
Sighing;
Psychotic nutter makes sense at last!

Pause,
Applause,
Snores;
She realizes, for the moment, her terror has subsided.

She sleeps the sleep of the heavily sedated.

Morn,
Is born,

To scorn;
Another day refreshes the worries of yesteryear.


## SOCIOLOGICAL RESEARCH No 1

Are you heterosexual, James?
Are you an out and proud heterosexual?
And will you hit me for asking?


## AN ANALYSIS OF MALE HETEROSEXUAL DEFENCE MECHANISMS

It's funny, you know,
Being a Gay man,
Talking to heterosexuals,
Well mainly men actually;
When you talk about sex,
And whom you fancy,
Or who fancies you,
Or who fancies who,
Or jealousy,
Or your unfaithful, ignorant, annoying and beautiful ex-lover,
Or what your first crush was like,
Or the heterosexual men who occasionally dabble,
Or the young man, the teenager still at school,
Bravely standing up for his love rights,
Or anything else really,
They cut you dead.

# FIRST BOOK

Silence.

Then talk about sport, TV, work, music,
And, after quite a while,
What women they angrily fancy.

It's funny, you know,
Being a Gay man,
Talking to heterosexuals,
Well mainly men actually;
When you talk about sex,

Because if the men are attracted to the women,
And if the women don't then give them their all,
Then the men feel betrayed and get angry.

It's funny, you know,
Being a Gay man,
Talking to heterosexuals,
Well mainly men actually;
When you talk about sex.


## SELF-INFLICTED

I'm a middle aged fool.
I can't read anything without my glasses,
Struggle to hear conversations in the pub,
Takes me five minutes to remember anyone's
name,
Skin the texture of uncooked pastry;
Still chasing twenty two year olds,

I'll be worn out by breakfast!

## IMPOSSIBLE DREAM

Every night
I dream of the same thing:
Of picking up a man
On the number 17 bus,
Taking him home,
And both of us,
Perfectly sober.

## FEEDBACK

Feedback – Feed plus Back,

Feed: to give food, often pertaining to animals or children. Food item for livestock, e.g. chickenfeed.

Back – to return, rear, not the front, e.g. out the back.

Feedback – to return food. To feed the one that fed you. Sometimes pertaining to children, e.g. "I'll eat one of yours. Now you eat one of mine." But not pertaining to animals.

# FIRST BOOK

## CLEANSING

In middle age,
When not wearing ones spectacles,
The World takes on a blurry, unfocussed quality,
Not unlike taking, or not taking,
Certain drugs.


## 2004 SYMPTOMS AND REFLECTIONS

More people take Prozac than voted in Pop Idol.
More people, many more, said to their Doctor,
"I am depressed, distressed, miserable and grey,"
Than hit the phone, hit the txt, jumped up and
down and sighed.
Maybe more people do not like themselves than
get excited by Robbie?

What value is there in comparing Will and Gareth
and Girls Aloud
To sub-clinical depression?

"Maybe we should talk more?" Proclaimed The
Samaritans on their poster.
Depression, Girls Aloud, Will Young, Txt,
The inherent competitiveness of Capitalism,
The impossibility of providing enough effective
counsellors,
The absolute need to lie in most job interviews
*(Yes, dear interviewer, seeing as you ask, the
biggest problem I would face, if I got this job,*

*would be being so excited that I would find it hard
to sleep at night!),*
The restructuring of society to prevent human
beings hating themselves,
The absolutely essential need for an Anarcho-
Socialist, Communist, Ecotopean revolution,
Girls Aloud, Will Young, Gareth Gates:
To talk, yes indeed, but about what?


## OBJECT RELATIONS THEORY

Between the useless and the stupid
Lies Object Relations Theory;
But objects, as explained by school book
grammar,
Cannot be stupid,
And people, have desire, desiring, i.e. free will,
And are not objects,
Except in the eye of the labeller,
Who, finding their will differs from certain others
Resort to labels of outstanding simplicity.
This momentarily results in a heightened sense of
power,
Immediately followed by an sense of frustration,
And then anger, or possibly rage.
Thus, most of the problems of the world
Can be explained without reference to either
Freud or Marx,
A triumph of intellectual simplicity
That will be endlessly commented on by the
intellectual community.

# FIRST BOOK

## BEEP-BEEP BEEP-BEEP

Wouldn't it be nice
If alarm clocks said,
"Hello sweetie, you asked me to make sure you
were up,
Doing anything nice today?"
And then, when you press the snooze button,
Said, "Have a nice snooze, I'll be back in ten
minutes,"
And in ten minutes time it said,
"Hello sweetie, are you ready to get up yet?"
Then, if you press it again, said,
"You can always switch me off and go back to
sleep if you like?"
Politely paused, and then said, "O.K. I'll be back in
ten minutes."
Wouldn't it be nice?


## LETTER POEM No 1

Dearest You

Growing lettuce,
I am gardening for money.
Pruning roses, clearing leaves,
I don't earn enough money to live on,
Perhaps I will if I try hard enough?
Though not in the dead of winter.

*John Hoggett*

My stepmother is in Devon,
I haven't spoken to her for fifteen years.
I wrote to her last year, she wrote back.
I didn't read the letter – too frightened.

I had a crush on you once.
Now you go walking by the river with a guy called
Ryan,
I am bitter, but not about you,
Just about life.

The climate is changing,
Human beings are killing themselves – slowly, but
not very slowly.
I have been asked to do workshops in schools,
I hope to inspire revolutionary spirit amongst
seventeen year olds.
No very likely,
Not enough to have much impact on climate
change.

A not very close friend had ECT last week
(That's where Doctors and Nurses induce an
epileptic seizure in your head
In the belief that they are saving a life
Because they cannot think of anything else to help
severely depressed people.
Not that they tried much,
Apart from locking you in a fucking boring hospital
ward
And doing "observations" on you).

# FIRST BOOK

I have had a poem published in a book called,
"This Is Madness."
It beautifully illustrates the theme
Of non-directive counselling with people
experiencing psychosis.
I'm good at it.
I enjoy it.
I liked my beautiful, psychotic friend, Marcus
Before he went out on the street
And thumped my friend Siren;
Mistaking her for a Devil or something.

I went to see my father and his wife,
Third wife actually.
I went with my brother a couple of months ago.
My father was really boring.
He ignored me and talked at my brother about
food.
He is eighty.
I hadn't seen him for years.
My father and I haven't got on since my
stepmother left him twenty-five years ago.

This is poetry, but not as we know it Jim;
Poetry, but not as we know it.

On Friday I go to Wallingford to perform poetry.
If I were really making a living as a gardener I
wouldn't go.
I would stay at home and promote my business.

*John Hoggett*

Yesterday my friend Chris phoned to say he was
going to Soho to pick up men.
I wonder if he succeeded?
Probably not.
My friend Nick and I discussed chatting people up
at bus stops.
He succeeded once,
I never have.

The neighbours are not talking to me.
I am not talking to the neighbours.
Perhaps this is for the best?

I have gone out in the dead of night
And graffitied, "Gay is Great!"
To balance out, "Ashley is Gay," that was already
there.
Next week I am going to put, "Batty is Best,"
To balance, "Ashley is Batty."
I don't suppose Ashley is best pleased.

I could go on like this forever,
But I will stop and post this letter.

Is this poetry, but not as we know it Jim?
Is this poetry, but not as we know it?

Lightning Source UK Ltd.
Milton Keynes UK
UKOW04f1521100316

269979UK00001B/2/P

9 781847 473806